Sally Collings is the author of So
Positive (2009). Sally worked in b
twenty years, dividing her time bet
Now based in Brisbane and a moth
writer and editor, specialising in life stories and inspirational
writing of all kinds.

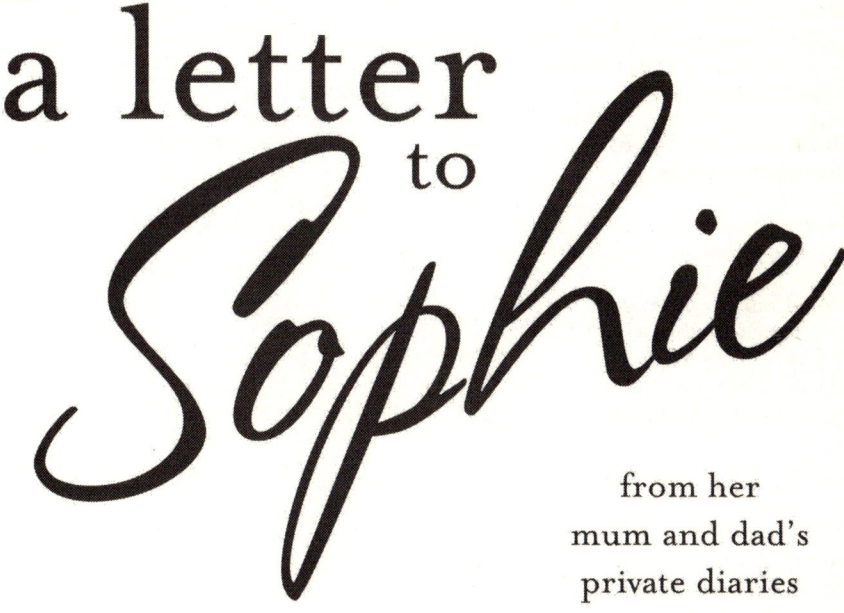

from her
mum and dad's
private diaries

CAROLYN MARTIN & RON DELEZIO
with SALLY COLLINGS

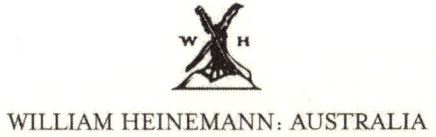

WILLIAM HEINEMANN: AUSTRALIA

A William Heinemann book
Published by Random House Australia Pty Ltd
Level 3, 100 Pacific Highway, North Sydney NSW 2060
www.randomhouse.com.au

First published by William Heinemann Australia in 2009

Copyright © Carolyn Martin and Ron Delezio 2009

The moral right of the authors has been asserted.

All rights reserved. No part of this book may be reproduced or transmitted by any person or entity, including internet search engines or retailers, in any form or by any means, electronic or mechanical, including photocopying (except under the statutory exceptions provisions of the Australian *Copyright Act 1968*), recording, scanning or by any information storage and retrieval system without the prior written permission of Random House Australia.

Addresses for companies within the Random House Group can be found at
www.randomhouse.com.au/offices.

National Library of Australia
Cataloguing-in-Publication Entry

    Martin, Carolyn.
    A letter to Sophie/Carolyn Martin and Ron Delezio.

ISBN: 978 1 74166 673 1 (pbk).

    Delezio, Sophie.
    Martin, Carolyn – Diaries.
    Delezio, Ron – Diaries.
    Children with disabilities – Care – New South Wales – Biography.
    Burns and scalds in children – New South Wales – Biography.
    Children – Wounds and injuries – New South Wales – Biography.
    Parents of children with disabilities – New South Wales – Diaries.

    Other authors/contributors: Delezio, Ron.

    305.9083

Cover design by Christabella Designs
Cover photographs © Elizabeth Alnutt, www.elizabethphotography.com.au
'I said a prayer for you today', on p. 25, reproduced by kind permission of Frank J. Zamboni.
Internal design by Melanie Fedderson/www.i2i.com.au
Typeset in 12/16 pt Sabon by Midland Typesetters, Australia
Printed and bound by Griffin Press, South Australia

Random House Australia uses papers that are natural, renewable and recyclable products and made from wood grown in sustainable forests. The logging and manufacturing processes are expected to conform to the environmental regulations of the country of origin.

10 9 8 7 6 5 4 3

To all who have journeyed with us, thank you. This book is for you. To those families still on the journey, I wish you well and Godspeed in your recovery and that of your child. In particular, this book is dedicated to Dr Peter Hayward, who gave us the precious gift of hope.

Carolyn Martin

To my beautiful wife, Carolyn, who has been a tower of strength, love and consistency to my family and me. To my son, Mitchell, who has also suffered so much and will continue to suffer the side effects of his sister's plight for the rest of his life. And to our dear daughter, Sophie, who has shown our family and so many millions of people around the world the power of love and positive thinking and perseverance. I am a different man because of the lessons life has taught me.

Ron Delezio

contents

foreword by Danny Green — ix

preface: **why we wrote this book** — xi

introduction — 1

    chapter one: **a bubble of pain** — 9

    chapter two: **making rainbows** — 34

    chapter three: **the price of innocence** — 51

    chapter four: **out of Intensive Care** — 67

    chapter five: **under pressure** — 83

    chapter six: **'I do not want to lose her'** — 97

    chapter seven: **withdrawal** — 117

    chapter eight: **turning the corner** — 132

    chapter nine: **one hundred days** — 144

    chapter ten: **Sophie is three** — 156

    chapter eleven: **Sophie's legs** — 171

    chapter twelve: **days of progress** — 185

    chapter thirteen: **exit strategy** — 205

    chapter fourteen: **'we're lucky'** — 219

    chapter fifteen: **going home** — 234

    chapter sixteen: **lightning strikes twice** — 249

    chapter seventeen: **the long haul** — 269

who's who — 281

medical terms and abbreviations — 286

acknowledgements — 288

foreword

Like most people, I became aware of Sophie Delezio in late 2003 by way of the tragic news story informing us of the horror crash at her day-care centre. A short time later, I was asked to donate a piece of memorabilia for a benefit night to raise money to assist the Delezio family with the crippling costs of her hospital care. I had no hesitation in offering my assistance, and Ron contacted me personally to thank me. After that, Ron and I formed our friendship together.

In April 2006, I asked the Delezio family if Sophie would do me the honour of carrying the Australian flag into the ring with me for my big fight against Anthony Mundine at Aussie Stadium. A week after we spoke about it, Sophie was involved in another shocking life-threatening accident, and the horror and pain for Sophie and her family unfolded once again.

I went to visit Sophie in Intensive Care, where she was in a coma. I spoke to her as if she was awake, and when I asked her to shake my hand, incredibly, she raised her hand and smiled! Ron and I both had tears in our eyes. It was a moment I will never forget. That little girl was going through more pain and torture than anyone could possibly fathom, and she still had the guts to raise her hand and smile.

When the boxing match came around on 17 May, Ron carried the Aussie flag on Sophie's behalf, wearing a photograph of her big, beautiful, smiling face on his T-shirt, and her spirit was with us all that night. The Delezio family are a very special unit.

People often ask me who my hero is and who inspires me as a fighter. My answer is simple: Sophie Delezio. I have had a lot of painful injuries throughout my career, but they are like stubbing your toe compared to the hell that Sophie Delezio has endured. I have never seen a human being with so much resilience and courage, and the toughness Sophie has displayed is nothing short of superhuman. I believe that we, as a country, should put her face on one of our coins, to remind us all of one little girl's determination to survive and what it truly means to never give up.

Sophie Delezio: a true Aussie battler.

Danny Green
Former WBA light heavyweight world champion and Olympian

preface
why we wrote this book

We have met people as young as five who have been positively affected by hearing Sophie's story. To many, it has given hope, strength, inspiration – and, importantly, an understanding of what people go through in dealing with a medical condition, the hospital system, rehabilitation and the sometimes complex challenges that life can throw your way.

We have written this book to give an insight into the roller coaster of emotions experienced by both patients and their families, to put a very real face on a picture that for many is hard to imagine, and to say thanks again to the teams that helped to get us in and out of the front doors of two hospitals. I wanted these diaries to capture Sophie's life during these dark days for her to read when she was ready, or, if they were to become a record of her last days or weeks or months, for Mitchell to have a permanent testament to the sister he had lost.

Looking at the diaries today, I have to say that they mean even more, reflecting as they do just how far Sophie and Mitchell and those who have journeyed with us have come, how we all change with life's chances, and what joy there is in the simple things. It is the simple things that can make a day truly special.

Carolyn Martin

We first decided to release this book to give the community a true understanding of what people go through when a tragedy hits their own family: the highs and lows, the depression and the tears that can only be imagined by those who have never experienced the near loss of their child.

Five years on from Sophie's first accident, I had never read Carolyn's diaries, let alone referred back to my own notes. Reading them after that time brought back the feelings of sadness and fear, as well as love and faith, which was tested on a daily basis. I remember saying to myself *how could these people continue dealing with this situation every day, through four months of uncertainty*, before realising that I was reading my own notes.

This book is truly a tribute to all of the mothers and fathers and friends who have spent what seems like a lifetime offering love and positivity to their child without thinking of themselves. It is also a tribute to the members of the medical profession who wear their hearts on their sleeves, seeing little ones continue to live or die during the daily course of their jobs. I hope that what we have seen and experienced will never be repeated, but I know full well that it is a journey that will be re-enacted time and time again for thousands of families. I hope that our story can make a difference to the way in which people support their community and the individuals in it, and to the way they support our charity, the Day of Difference Foundation, so that critically injured kids and their families can benefit from their generosity. A portion of the profits from this book will be going to the Day of Difference Foundation.

Ron Delezio

introduction

Sophie Delezio has faced death twice before the age of six. When she was only two and a half years old, she was trapped under a burning car that had crashed into her childcare centre. She suffered burns to eighty-five per cent of her body before being rescued. In hospital, she was subjected to multiple amputations and skin grafts on her long road to recovery. Then, two and a half years later, lightning struck a second time. Soon after her fifth birthday, Sophie was hit by a car on a pedestrian crossing. Again, she held onto life by a slender thread. Her irrepressible smile and sheer determination have captured hearts throughout Australia and the wider world.

Many of us first came to know Sophie on 15 December 2003. Initially, we didn't know her name, but we knew the facts: that a car had careered into the Roundhouse Childcare Centre at Fairlight, on Sydney's Northern Beaches; that two children had been trapped under the car and severely burnt, while others had been treated for minor burns and shock; and, finally, that those two children, Sophie Delezio and Molly Wood, had been taken to the Burns Unit at the Children's Hospital at Westmead, where their lives hung in the balance.

Accidents, by definition, should never happen. This one in particular seemed unthinkable. Ten days before Christmas; preschoolers having their afternoon nap; a car so out of control that it flew through a window. Unbelievable that it happened, unbelievable that no one was killed.

During the days that followed, the wider community watched and waited for news of Molly and Sophie. The hospital switchboard jammed with calls from the public. If heaven has a switchboard, it was running hot too, as there was little any of us could do but pray. Days stretched into weeks; it seemed these two little girls were not leaving us any time soon, but it was months before even that was certain.

Sophie's parents, Ron and Carolyn, are intimately acquainted with that count of days. This book is based on the diaries they kept after Sophie's accident, in which they number the days after the event that divided their lives as cleanly as a scalpel: there was life before the accident, and life after. Nothing would ever be the same again. Ron explained to me the abruptness of the shift: 'I remember being with Sophie [in the hospital] around two or three o'clock in the morning and there was a woman there whose daughter had a brain tumour. She came up to me and she told me how much she prayed for Sophie and how much she cared about what was going on with her. I turned to her and said, "I should be saying the same thing to you, because your daughter's drastically ill as well." She thanked me but she said, "Your situation is different. You're going through a tragedy. We're going through a sickness." It was only recently I realised what she was talking about: with us it was that instant, that second, from one side to the other, whereas with her it was a gradual process in which she had time to learn how to cope with the situation.'

Keeping a diary did not come naturally to Ron. As he said, 'Our lawyer asked us to keep notes of what was going on in the hospital system, what was going on with Sophie and ourselves – mainly for legal reasons, just in case we needed to talk about our experiences in court for certain claims. It was pretty hard for me because I'd never written a diary before. I didn't know how. What sort of format do you put it in? Do you do it by date? Do you do it by time? Do you say, "Now I'm walking down the stairs"? I just didn't have a clue. So I asked a lot of our friends and went from there.' Ron only began keeping regular diary notes seven weeks after Sophie's accident; his entries for the days before that were written later, when he read through the hospital case notes on Sophie's treatment.

For Carolyn, it seemed second nature to keep a diary. She had kept one in the past – not every day, but to record significant moments and turning points. Soon after the accident (and before the legal considerations were raised), she asked Catherine, Ron's daughter from a previous marriage, to buy her a journal so that she could pour out her thoughts and emotions in its pages. That first diary became a 'letter to Sophie', in which Carolyn told Sophie about her hopes and prayers for her, the visitors who loved her, the public support for her, the good days and bad days, the doctors and nurses and what they were doing to help save her life. Six weeks after the accident, Carolyn started a new diary that was intended for her eyes only. In it, she wrote out her fears, her frustration and anger.

Together, the letter to Sophie, Carolyn's journal and Ron's journal build up a picture of how the family got through each day.

Before Sophie's accident, a significant event for the Delezio family was moving house, or a new business opportunity, or a birthday. Ron was self-employed; Carolyn was in the process of buying a rental-management company. It had not been easy for them to have children, so Mitchell, aged four, and Sophie, aged two, were the light of their lives. Ron's parents, brothers and sisters also lived in Sydney, but Carolyn's family was scattered across the globe, with her parents in New Zealand, sister Ann-Louise in France and brother Gregory in the US. The Delezio family enjoyed an active social life. Their weekends were busy with barbecues and casual get-togethers with a wide circle of friends.

They will never know that simple, easy life again. But you could say that it is because of the very nature of the Delezios' pre-accident life, their way of looking at the world, the tight support of friends and family, that they were able to save Sophie's life – and their own.

Ron had long believed in the power of a positive outlook in strengthening the body and the mind. 'We purposely didn't cry in front of Sophie at all. We wanted to leave all those emotions outside the room so that she only dealt with positive thoughts. We did all our crying outside. We didn't want her to think that we were being affected in that way. She had enough to worry about herself.'

Carolyn was a firm advocate of alternative therapies, including reiki, the Japanese healing practice in which energy is used to assist the patient's natural healing ability. Practitioners say that reiki harmonises the energy pathways, allowing life force to flow in a natural, healthy way. It is often used together with shiatsu massage, another traditional Japanese practice that is based on the principles of energy and meridians. For Carolyn, it was natural to help her critically ill daughter by using reiki and visualisation techniques alongside mainstream medicine, calling on alternative therapies as an adjunct to an extensive and long-term program of painkillers and sedatives administered by the hospital. The Delezios stopped short of giving Sophie any herbal remedies, as they decided to let Western medicine take the lead in Sophie's treatment.

They were never the kind of people who shied away from asking for help when help was available, Ron said. 'It didn't take us long after the accident before we started to see the social worker and some psychiatrists, learning how to deal with the situation. It reminded me of when we were just married. It was such a big deal – Carolyn had never been married before; I had been married before. We were madly in love, but it's such a risky thing to do. Around six months after we married, we started going to a marriage-guidance counsellor because we wanted to see that we were doing the right things and make sure we were getting all the right advice. We didn't want it not to work. And this was the same situation here.'

Ron and Carolyn's tight network of friends and family, in addition, helped them to cope with their tragedy in ways too numerous to detail, from forming rosters to sit with Sophie and look after Mitchell, to bringing meals, to helping them deal with the media, such as by sending text-message updates on Sophie's condition.

'We're very lucky with how things came together in terms of Grandma and Grandpa [Martin] coming over from New Zealand and taking care of Mitchell,' Ron told me. 'We knew it was the right thing to have Mitchell go to day care during the day just so he'd have some normality in his life. Also to take the pressure off us having to worry about him, because we were desperately worried about Mitchell as well, but we needed all the time we had to focus on what was happening with Sophie. There were so many different medical people we needed to talk to regarding her condition, let alone having to deal with our own emotions and our own problems, such as sleep deprivation. With me, there was also depression setting in. The sleep deprivation was making me hallucinate and not see straight at all, but then to see people with other kids walking around – I just cried all the time and I couldn't stop. I was feeling that I was going to be no good to anyone if I continued, so I went to the psychologist to get advice. They put me on antidepressants, and I must admit it didn't take long before I started to feel a little bit normal again, if there ever was going to be any normality in our life. It just allowed me to get on with caring for Sophie and Carolyn and Mitchell more than I was able to before.'

Above all, the Delezio family sought strength and comfort in God through this time. 'Every day, we said prayers with Sophie,' recalled Ron. 'I personally said prayers to Mary MacKillop [the Roman Catholic nun who co-founded the Sisters of St Joseph of the Sacred Heart in Australia in 1866] as well, holding Sophie's hand. We knew the doctors were doing everything they could. We were stuck with just holding her hand – the one hand she has left that's complete – and hoping and praying for the best.'

By 2006, Sophie's family were starting to see the light at the end of the tunnel. Ron and Carolyn had just sat down with Sophie's plastic surgeon, Peter Hayward, and scheduled a break from the relentless rounds of operations that their daughter needs in order to repair her skin and accommodate her growing body. Then, on 5 May, Sophie was hit by a car on a pedestrian crossing. Her injuries were again horrific and potentially fatal.

It is a testament to the kind of people that they are that, rather than being consumed with anger and despair, Ron and Carolyn said to themselves, 'We know what to do. We know how to deal with this,' and plunged once again into the world of emergency surgery, a barrage of media attention, meal rosters and pain management.

Just over five years on from Sophie's first life-changing accident, Ron and Carolyn offer up their private diaries to public view. They have always taken the attitude that if their story can help one other child with burns, or one family with a critically ill son or daughter, or someone waiting for their own surgery, then something good will have come from their own tragedy. In the course of turning their journals into a book, the Delezios sat down and read through the mountainous case notes kept by the Children's Hospital at Westmead and Sydney Children's Hospital at Randwick about their daughter's care.

Ron reflected on that process: 'I can't believe I'm sitting here after all this time looking over a copy of the clinical notes, seeing the thousands and thousands of pages of things that were done to Sophie – operations, procedures, medicines, medications, dressings, amputations – and taking my mind back to when that first accident happened.

'To look back now after five years and see what Sophie's gone through, see what our family has gone through, our trials and tribulations as parents, as husband and wife: Carolyn as a mother was faultless, all the way through; as a father, I struggled at different times with depression and not knowing what to do, trying to be strong, being in denial some of that time as well.

'Right from the start, I remember not being able to believe that this sort of thing had happened to my family, to my little girl. She's such a baby. To think that she was in any sort of pain was just so distressing for me and for Carolyn and for Mitchell. And to see her go through these awful operations one at a time, the things that she had to go through every day, just makes me feel that she is superhuman, to be able to tolerate all these things.

'And we wondered, were we making the right decision? It's all right now in hindsight to look back and say we were – we believe we were, because we still don't really know what the rest of her life is going to be like. But, back in those times, we were asking ourselves, is she going to live a life of pain, a life of people putting her down, a life of not being able to get any jobs or struggling to make friends or find the right schooling? We didn't know all these things back then and we fought for everything we've got.

'I remember Carolyn and I sometimes both going into the operating theatre with Sophie. The rules were that there was only one parent allowed at a time and we broke those rules a number of times for certain operations. The other times, when it was Carolyn's turn, I remember how much I hated being left behind, how much I wanted to be with Carolyn and to be the last person to see Sophie before she went through the operation. If something had happened to Sophie and she hadn't come out of theatre alive, I would have felt so cheated not to have been the last person in our family to see her.'

Sophie is a fighter. She is still here, sparkling with life and energy and bringing joy to all who meet her. How did she survive? There's no one answer to that question. There are thousands of answers, as many as people who held her hand or dressed her wounds or lit a candle or said a prayer. And a large part of the answer lies with Ron and Carolyn and Mitchell, who never left her side.

Sally Collings

chapter one
a bubble of pain

One phone call. That is all it takes to change a life. Before that call on 15 December 2003, the Delezio family were busy, happy, healthy – normal, if there is such a thing. After it, they have a horribly injured daughter clinging to life, a barrage of media attention, decisions to make about living and dying. For them, there is no gentle easing into illness or preparation for disaster. And, for a long time, none of it seems quite real.

Ron's journal, Monday 15 December 2003
At 2.20 pm, I had a phone call from the police saying that Sophie was involved in an accident and telling me to go to the Roundhouse Childcare Centre. On the way, I heard the news on the radio about the crash. I sped to the Roundhouse to find ambulances and fire engines all over the place. I was in a panic, still not knowing what had really happened. I ran the last two hundred metres, as the road was blocked off. When I arrived,

I saw kids all over the grass, a car on its side, smoke everywhere, fire engines, ambulances, paramedics, parents screaming and crying, and I just didn't know what to feel at all. I couldn't see Sophie. Someone [a police officer] told me that Sophie had been taken to hospital [the Royal North Shore Hospital in St Leonards] but they couldn't tell me her condition. They said that I needed to go to the hospital quick smart. I started running back to the car and the police officer caught up with me and said, 'No, no, you're not driving. Come with me.' I was crying and getting more upset, not knowing what was wrong. There were no sirens but the police driver was moving faster than the speed limit. Halfway there, around Mosman, I received a phone call from the hospital asking where we were. I said Mosman and he said to get to the hospital asap. I have never been so scared in my life. I rang Caro and told her to go straight to the hospital and I would meet her there. I just burst into tears, thinking *this is real; it's not just a movie.*

When I arrived at the hospital, I went directly to Emergency, where I found about twenty doctors and nurses around the bed. I met up with Caro and then we had a meeting with the doctors, who explained what had happened. We were asked if we would like to see Sophie. I said yes. All I can remember were Sophie's little toes, charred black, sticking out from the bandages. She was covered in foil from her head to the ends of her legs. So we gave Sophie a kiss on the little area that we could. The local priest came and gave Sophie his blessing; it was like watching a movie with someone getting the last rites.

We were then told that they had the helicopter ready to take Sophie to the Children's Hospital at Westmead but they had to wait until she was stable. The time finally came and Sophie was ready to be transported to Westmead. I agreed to go with her: I thought if a decision had to be made about Sophie it should be up to me to make that decision. I felt as though I needed to be the rock of the family.

It was all so surreal at the time. We weren't screaming; we were crying, but for me it was controlled crying because I really didn't believe that something so serious could happen to us or to our baby girl. But it could. It was happening right then and there, and it was the beginning of the rest of our lives, I suppose.

We were in the lift going to the eighth floor (the roof). It stopped on the seventh floor as we didn't have a pass to go higher. They found a security guard, who swiped his card in the elevator, and off we went to the eighth floor. They showed me the procedure for the flight and I was given a helmet and told where to sit, with Sophie lying on the bed nearby. It took six and a half minutes from take-off to landing at Westmead.

Sophie was taken to theatre and I met up with Caro [who was driven to the Children's Hospital in a police car] and some friends. We held each other close and I could feel Caro's body almost collapsing in my arms. I don't know how many hours Sophie was away. We spoke to the Intensive Care Unit [ICU] doctors, chaplains and social workers about Sophie's condition. The right side of Caro's face and her legs were going into convulsions. We took Caro to Westmead Hospital, next door, where she was given some diazepam. They believe it was due to the anxiety of the situation; they were a bit concerned that it was a stroke at the time, induced by what had happened. She was away for around seven hours. I felt so alone, with so much pain and agony.

We were ushered into a meeting room and asked to wait. The first doctor we met who came through the door was in tears, and I just couldn't understand – couldn't believe – that these medical people in Intensive Care, going through these situations all the time, would be taking it so hard. I suppose it made us feel the severity of what Sophie was going through. We were told by the ICU doctors that Sophie may not make it and that eighty-five per cent of her body had third-degree burns. Soph was taken back to bed four, where I saw her charred little feet again sticking out of the bandages. I remember the day

a bubble of pain

before holding Sophie and playing with her toes. They were so beautiful and soft.

We were given a bedroom in ICU to sleep in, and I think we dozed off around 4 am.

Ron's journal, Tuesday 16 December 2003
Around eleven o'clock, they decided to relieve some of the pressure in Sophie's abdomen. Her whole body was swelling up to twice the size of her original body. Because the skin will only stretch so far, it all gets pushed in and it was putting pressure on her insides – her heart, her lungs, her liver, all her internal organs. What they did was they opened Sophie's whole gut out and sucked up around 800 ml of fluid from her insides. This procedure was called a laparotomy. They also did a cut – a release – all the way down Sophie's left- and right-hand sides. They just got a knife and cut all the way through her flesh – probably about half an inch to an inch deep – to relieve some of the pressure on the internal organs. They then sewed a clear plastic bag around the open wound in her stomach and brought that up to a point above her bed, where they put a ring in the bag and hung it from a tripod. Even though they sucked the fluid out, because of Sophie's increase in size they couldn't put the ends of the stomach back together. So you'd go and see Sophie and you'd see her intestines, all her internal organs . . .

By this time, it was around seven at night and we'd been there for twenty-four hours. We were getting pretty tired but still pretty focused on what was going on. Sophie had a few infections from the laparotomy site and from the side, the enterotomy site. There started to be oozing. I'm starting to panic again; it was almost midnight and I was starting to freak about what was going on with Sophie, the seriousness of her condition. We need to go away from Sophie's side to speak to someone. I'm getting increasingly nervous about whether she's being taken care of properly. Carolyn's still having panic attacks and is mentioning a tingling sensation down the right side of her body. There always seem to be five or six pumps pumping something into Sophie: there was platelets, there was blood, there was antibiotics, albumin – I'd never seen so many different types of medicine going into someone in one go.

Ron's journal, Wednesday 17 December 2003
We had Mitchell in again today. He would only go as far as the door; he wouldn't go near Sophie. He was so scared about what was going on, you could only imagine what was going through his mind at the time. He kept on asking questions about what was happening with Sophie. Considering he is only four and a half, we have to be very careful how to talk to Mitchell. But we had to tell him the truth, we had to tell him about the accident and about the burns.

We had a meeting with Dr Liz Henderson and Dr Adrien Falkov – they're the psych registrars at the hospital. We spoke with them about our feelings. Carolyn's always very good in discussing her feelings and talked about how it feels like a bit of a roller coaster going on, and how the uncertainty of it all is really hurting us both, and a feeling of hopelessness and sometimes guilt. I keep on feeling the need to cry but I feel I need to stay controlled all the time. They keep on saying you're going to need to let it out, but the time's not right and I don't know when the time will be right.

They're talking now about closing her abdomen tomorrow; what a relief that would be.

Catherine Delezio, Ron's daughter from a previous marriage, gave Carolyn a blank journal in which to record her thoughts and feelings following Sophie's accident. This is the book that Carolyn used to write her letter to Sophie.

> Dear Caro,
> I give you this journal in the hope that it brings some release to your pain. I wish it was a gift rather than a tool to your own survival through this very hard time in your life. Caro, you are such a wonderful mother to your two beautiful children and Soph knows that. I hope you understand that she is as strong as this because you made her that way. I pray that she hears your and the world's prayers. I am here for you.
> Love, Catherine

Letter to Sophie, Thursday 18 December 2003
Miracle 1:
A burning car was lifted by your rescuers.
Miracle 2:
You sustained no head, organ or spinal injuries.
Miracle 3:
Louise, a paediatrician, travelled with you to hospital. (Louise Northcott, Emergency department registrar, the Children's Hospital at Westmead.)
Miracle 4:
You survived the Careflight trip to Westmead. (Your NETS [medical retrieval] crew were Paul Crouchman and Wendy Bladwell.)

Princess, your lips were red today!
   What beautiful lips . . .
   And I kissed them.
   Since you arrived at hospital, you have had so much support from friends and family.

You are a miracle to have survived your serious injuries this long and I am so proud of you. My darling, we are taking just one hour at a time and you have survived your second serious operation since Monday afternoon's accident. You are still in critical condition and we hope and pray that you make it one more day.

We feel blessed that we have been given that chance since Monday.

You are a special, special girl and have touched so many hearts it is overwhelming. Your bravery and courage are an inspiration to me.

I love you so. x

(Uncle Greg arrived from the US today.)

Your special Paediatric Intensive Care Unit [PICU] nurses are:
– Irene Kopp
– Tricia Cummins
– Helenne Levy
– Angela Holden
– Kathryn McNamara
– Gemma Lowe
– Louise Jennings
– Bettina Kolker
– Amy Gaffey.

Courage
Hope
Trust
Faith
Compassion
Belief
Humour
Love

Ron's journal, Thursday 18 December 2003

Woke at 7 am after spending the first night in the parents' hostel, knowing that some of our friends are watching over our dear daughter; I felt comforted knowing that Sophie has such a large extended family that loves her. I'm anxious about Sophie's next chapter. I hope to God it stays positive in direction. I feel I am a better person – the person I have always wanted to be, even under these circumstances.

Sophie's swelling is starting to come down a bit. They've been unable to check her pupils: because of the swelling, her eyes are permanently closed. This is the first time they've been able to check them.

We had our first meeting with Sophie's plastic surgeon, Dr Hayward, just talking about possible outcomes. They're now talking about the need to amputate Sophie's right leg and her left foot. We're trying to take in all this information – it's just incredible. It still seems surreal that we're talking to the doctors about cutting something off our little baby.

During the day, we are told Sophie could be here for nine or ten months. I put it out of my mind quickly to move on to the duties of the day. Who could imagine that three days ago I had a beautiful, healthy daughter?

In Ron and Carolyn's journals, 'Day 1' equates to Friday 19 December, four days after Sophie's accident. Before this, death was imminent, minute by minute. In those first few days, the sheer magnitude of the decisions and emotions confronting them didn't allow time or energy for them to write anything down.

The most critical danger for Sophie now is infection. Without her skin to protect her, she is vulnerable to all the bugs and bacteria that come her way. Ironically, the very drugs used to combat infection are highly toxic and can lead to organ shutdown, so the longer a patient is without full skin coverage, the greater the risk of fatal infection or organ failure. It is the ultimate race against time.

Sophie has various lines going into her body to administer painkillers, deliver liquid feeds and check her blood – all essential for her, but any time something enters the body from outside it is a potential source of infection.

Letter to Sophie, Day 1, Friday 19 December 2003
I feel I have missed the beginning of this tale. On Monday, Dad rang and said you had been in an accident and were being taken to hospital. I jumped into the car and raced to Royal North Shore, ringing Linda [friend] on the way. Dad was being driven by the police. I arrived first and my life was forever changed.

You were critical and had to be stabilised before the Westpac flight to Westmead but your life was saved by the quick actions of Louise – the paediatrician who held your hand after the accident and travelled to hospital with you – and the staff at the Royal North Shore.

Linda travelled with me in the police car to Westmead; you travelled with Dad in the helicopter. Our friends Wayne, Carolyn, James, Maree, Linda, Beth, Lee were with us at this time. The Delezio family came. Auntie Ann-Louise arrived from France today.

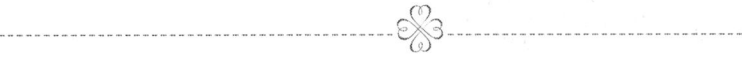

Letter to Sophie, Day 2, Saturday 20 December 2003
Today, princess, you lose your legs, but if it gives us a chance to have you with us for more time that's all that matters – we will get through the rest.

Our friends Mandy, Louise, Katrina, John [Miller, Katrina's husband] and Dave have been an amazing support; you have not been alone since you arrived here. You have guardian angels everywhere and people praying around the world.

a bubble of pain

There are presents and flowers from people we don't know arriving to give you support.

We are blessed with another day to tell you how much we love you, to sing songs to you, to read stories to you and just to be near you.

Ron's journal, Day 2, Saturday 20 December 2003
We had to say goodbye to Sophie this morning; she's going into theatre for a huge operation to remove both of her feet. It's unbelievable feeling so completely useless. We can't do anything; we've just got to let our little girl go. What do they do with the feet? I don't know whether I should ask for them back so we can bury them. All we can ask the doctors is that they bring back as much of our little girl as possible, and we show them a photo of Sophie before the accident so they know what she looked like before.

The operation took around three hours. Around one o'clock, Sophie was back in Intensive Care.

Letter to Sophie, Day 3, Sunday 21 December 2003
At Concord Hospital Burns Unit, they have a special treatment, which has been applied to your back. Peter Hayward, your plastic surgeon, has been in consultation with them and they are treating your injuries as best they can. Indirectly, we have seen the benefit of the knowledge gathered to help the Bali bombing victims.

I LOVE YOU!

Letter to Sophie, Day 4, Monday 22 December 2003
Your second big operation today: forty per cent of the dead

skin was removed from your body and you made it through – what joy!

Oh, my princess, my hurt is so intense but my love is even more so, and if I can pour that over you to help you get better I will! I would do anything to have you well.

Today, your pupils responded. You are our special girl and we love you so!

Ron's journal, Day 4, Monday 22 December 2003
I just feel that I need to ask as many questions of the doctors as I can. It's upsetting for me to ask those questions, but probably a bit more upsetting for Carolyn. She keeps on leaving the bedside as it's getting a bit too hard for her, which I can understand.

I'm starting to realise how important nurses are, especially in Intensive Care: it's actually twenty-four-hours-a-day care with two nurses on twelve-hour shifts. From the beginning of the shift to the end of the shift, they're totally focused on every little adjustment Sophie needs to be comfortable. I don't know how they do it; there's no way in the world I'd be able to do that. These nurses are like doctors.

Letter to Sophie, Day 5, Tuesday 23 December 2003
I'm so scared to go in your room for fear of infection – for fear of losing you . . .

Today, I went to Mitchell's school Christmas party and I spent some time with him at home. He misses you terribly and wants you home too.

You are running marathons twenty-four hours a day!

Love is a total power of being.

Love, like the colour of sunset, sheds an aura of beauty wherever you look.

a bubble of pain

[Later.] 'Sensational' – from Dr Damian Marucci.

Peter Hayward says nothing will stay on your body that doesn't need to be there. Be strong, little girl.

Lucas's mum [Lucas was another Westmead patient] gave me a cross today from her mentor and friend, a monk. The cross has some of the timber from Jesus's cross in it. She asked me to put it on your tummy and say a prayer. We will do it again when you come out of the hospital operating room.

Beth brought blankie in today and put it on your bed; your breathing strengthened and went from twenty to thirty-five.

Katrina's prayer for Sophie

Strengthen our beautiful Sophie
O Lord, to do what she has to do
And bear what she has to bear
That accepting your healing gifts
Through the skill of surgeons and nurses
And the love that surrounds her
She may be restored to health
In this world
Through Jesus Christ our Lord
Amen

A Prayer for our Molly and Sophie

Guardian angel from heaven so bright
Watching beside me to lead me aright
Fold thy wings round me and guard me with love
Softly sing songs to me of heaven above
Amen
With all our love, The Roundhouse

Spoke with the hospital chaplain, Jan Donohoo; I do not want to become hardened and bitter through this journey.

Your beautiful face and shining spirit have touched so many lives.

I am holding your hand *every* minute of *every* day!

Today, I am going home to wrap Christmas presents with Mitchell to put under the tree. Mitchell has a special present for you, beautiful girl.

You are stable and it looks like you will start your grafts tomorrow.

You have a guardian angel who will take you wherever you need to go.

Things people can do to help:
– pray
– give blood
– donate to the burns units.

[Later.] You are my true champion and I love you so.

Mitchell's spirit is with you every day, my darling girl.

You had your first graft today and you did really, really well. And you are not on adrenaline – we are so proud of you.

You are A+ blood type.

Ron's journal, Day 5, Tuesday 23 December 2003
Around 5.30 pm: Sophie's come out of theatre. We're also told that the fingers on Sophie's right hand will have to be removed. All I could say to them was to leave as much as they can. I just can't stop feeling that there's more that I could be doing, or that we should be doing, or that the doctors should be doing. I suppose we're still questioning what they're going to do and whether they need to go that far. I suppose it's just a matter of not understanding how they work. We've been in Intensive Care for about eight days so far, and you wait to hear it: the bells and whistles go off, and doctors and nurses rush into certain areas of Intensive Care. I think we've already had around five children who haven't made it. It's just

incredible to think that your own child might be next. We've been told all the possibilities and they've asked us a couple of times already whether we should turn the machine off, talking about what Sophie's quality of life is likely to be, should we allow her to live in that sort of pain. How do you know what to do in these situations?

Letter to Sophie, Day 6, Wednesday 24 December 2003
You opened your eyes today!

Mitchell had a sleepover and a visit from Ronald McDonald. [The clown does tours of hospitals to visit sick children.] He was very concerned and wanted us to tell Ronald as soon as we saw his red shoes to 'Go away – Mitchell doesn't want to see you'. Maree had to leave a note by his door.

You open your eyes first for Peter Hayward, Daddy, Mummy and Santa and have been promised lots of jelly beans when you wake up.

You have a small infection at the moment and a little sore on your nose, but what joy I felt when I saw your beautiful, beautiful eyes. Jan said prayers to you and you opened your eyes. I said 'beautiful girl' and you opened your eyes.

You are my star – my guiding light.

Ron's journal, Day 6, Wednesday 24 December 2003
Scott and Caroline Wood, Molly's parents, are obviously going through exactly what we're going through. [Molly received burns to forty per cent of her body in the accident.] It's strange how it's a little bit of a relief to know someone who's going through something similar. Even though obviously we don't want them to suffer with their daughter, it gives us that connection, to know that someone knows how we're feeling. It's just so nice sometimes to be able to go downstairs and have

a bit of a chat with someone you know, even though we didn't know the Woods that well before.

We're getting a lot of help from John and Catherine, my children [aged thirty-two and twenty-six respectively at the time]. They always seem to be there, relieving us when we need them to. Catherine's spending a lot of time doing a complete night shift with Sophie; it's given me a bit of quiet time with Carolyn, just to lie in bed and talk to one another, and it's been refreshing to have that time together.

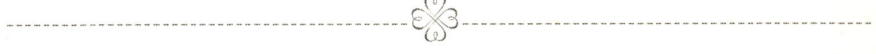

Letter to Sophie, Day 7, Thursday 25 December 2003
Happy Christmas, princess.

You are alert and talking – well, moving your lips, coughing and saying 'Mummy'.

I want you to know I am with you always and will never, ever let your hand go.

Catherine told me today that the first paramedic on the scene of the accident visited you today – he brought you a Christmas gift.

Well, my darling, I was with you in spirit today as I travelled home to be with Mitchell this morning so we could unwrap some presents and have a swim. Mitchell said as we drove back to Ronald McDonald House [accommodation for families of sick children at Australia's major women's and children's hospitals], 'Sometimes I visit you and sometimes you visit me.'

Arabella Miller
Little Arabella Miller
Had a furry caterpillar
First it walked upon her mother
Then upon her baby brother
They said 'Arabella Miller!
Take away your caterpillar!'

Actions
Finger like a caterpillar
Finger up one arm then the other
Hide hands behind back on last sentence

Just remember you are in my heart
I am in your heart
We may be apart
But we are always together inside
Because our hearts are joined
You are in me
And I am in you
Ann-Louise [Carolyn's sister]

Ron's journal, Day 7, Thursday 25 December 2003

Today is a pretty hard day, being Christmas Day. It's supposed to be a day when we're all happy and as a family, and here we are still battling for Sophie's life. Every time I look at Carolyn and see the stress on her face, it's just very hard for me to take, seeing someone you love being hurt so badly. Not only Sophie – I'm talking about Carolyn too. But there's no choice.

During the day, we had Santa Claus coming around the ward, showing a bit of cheer for the day. For me, it made me a bit sadder, I think. Just the same, we've got a photograph of Santa Claus near Sophie's bed.

It's happy Christmas to you, Sophie. We love you very much and we wish you weren't going through this.

Letter to Sophie, Day 8, Friday 26 December 2003

You have gone to theatre to have your dressings changed and

to see how your graft is. I sat in the chapel for quiet time and to reflect on your courage.

You are our brave, sweet princess and this morning when Daddy asked if you were his princess you nodded your head.

Our friend Chris Sharma has arrived from New Zealand to be a moral support to us all. Mitchell has asked what time you will be better. Messages arrive every day and we know prayers are being said in England, France, Italy, Austria, Malta, Germany, South Africa, USA, New Zealand. People who don't know you are touched by your story and bravery.

Jan said a prayer and Sue [Lucas's mum] lent her cross before you went to theatre – you are in very good hands.

I said a prayer for you today
And know God must have heard
I felt the answer in my heart
Although He spoke no word.

I didn't ask for wealth or fame
I knew you wouldn't mind
I asked Him to send treasures
Of a far more lasting kind.

I asked that He'd be near you
At the start of each new day
To grant you health and blessings
And friends to share your way.

I asked for happiness for you
In all things great and small
But it was for His loving care
I prayed the most of all.
  Frank J. Zamboni

Ron's journal, Day 8, Friday 26 December 2003
Sophie seems a lot more awake and alert and is responding to interaction; it makes us feel that there's a bit of hope now.

Most nights, we go back to our unit in the hospital [in Ronald McDonald House] and we have dinner with the Wood family. We sit down and have a few laughs now and then just to break the monotony of being so serious. I find it very strange that we can laugh when so many serious things are going on, but we've always been very social, happy people and I suppose if we didn't continue that, another part of our lives would have stopped.

Letter to Sophie, Day 9, Saturday 27 December 2003
The doctors, Peter Hayward and Damian, gave you ten out of ten. But I saw you in pain so I said to put it in a bubble and blow it away. We have to paint pictures in the mind, princess, to create a safe and happy place for you to be.

They are feeding you differently today so you can absorb more protein – this will help with the healing process.

I did a t'ai chi class in the park this morning while Chris Sharma took Dad for a walk around the river.

Ron's journal, Day 9, Saturday 27 December 2003
Because of all the infections that Sophie's got, she's having a lot of antibiotics pumped into her. The thing that kills most children with burns is infection. Her body temperature keeps going up and down; strangely enough, they treat that with just paracetamol at first. If it gets too high – we've had temperatures up into the forties – we go and get some ice from the ice machine in the next ward. Carolyn and I take it in shifts to get plastic bags and fill them full of ice and put them all around Sophie. At first, the nurse was doing it for us but we thought it best that she stay with Sophie and take care of her while we did it for her.

Letter to Sophie, Day 10, Sunday 28 December 2003
Today, I'm going to research pain-management techniques and products to use later for your grafts. I'm teaching everyone to encourage you to paint pictures in your mind, to take you to a happy, safe place where you like to be, to think of happy days and wonderful things that you like to do: slides, swings. Maybe I can teach you the notes on the piano. I want to teach you how to use your core energy to help heal your body.

Make shapes with the clouds, princess, as you look out the window.

You have a bit of a temperature so they will change your arterial line today.

Ron's journal, Day 10, Sunday 28 December 2003
We're staying in Ronald McDonald House at the moment. Over the Christmas break, a lot of the Oncology families go back home because there's no elective surgery. It feels like we're in a hotel after sleeping in the hostel: we've got a room for ourselves and a bathroom. It's not the best but it feels like a five-star hotel after what we've been used to: before Christmas we were sleeping next to beds and in chairs, or in the hospital's parents' hostel, which has got wire around the place, guards and no children allowed – it was an awful place. At Ronald McDonald House, there's a big family room with televisions and a big open-plan kitchen, people are talking to us and we're talking to other people – a bit of normality again.

We have a better understanding now of what's going on in the hospital system. When the nurses are talking about drugs and the doctors are talking about procedures, we understand what they're talking about. Because we're a part of the whole thing, they're acknowledging that by telling us everything they're doing and asking permission to do certain things. It's amazing that we can say, 'No, no, you've tried that before and

a bubble of pain

you can't do that because she had a reaction.' So we're starting to be a part of the medical team in a way.

Letter to Sophie, Day 11, Monday 29 December 2003
We told you that you are in hospital and sick, needing the nurses and doctors and Mummy and Daddy and yourself to help care for you. I told you that you have a yellow ball to hold in your tummy; its energy needs to spread to your legs, body and arms to help them get better.

You have an infection today and they may need to undress some of the bandages to help you cool down.

Hurray! You are breathing by yourself. You keep surprising everyone, my little princess.

Peter [Hayward] and Damian were called and you underwent a procedure to check your grafts, which were fine. Your temperature is down and you are stable.

Letter to Sophie, Day 12, Tuesday 30 December 2003
Every day, we walk into your room and give you energy from our hearts – another day on the roller coaster.

We squeeze your finger and you acknowledge with a squeeze.

You have had high temperatures for the last two and a half days but the ice packs today seem to keep things in check. Your temperature ranges from around 37 to 39.9 degrees, which is consistent. Ice cools your body.

You are doing deep-breathing exercises with me to relax you and are very good at it!

I am smothering you in white light filled with love from everybody. Therese [a friend of Katrina's] did a healing on you today to balance your electromagnetic field.

You receive beautiful messages and prayers from around the world and there is amazing fund-raising for you and Molly by the local community – Jeff [the purple Wiggle] attended the street party in Edwin Street [Fairlight].

Ron's journal, Day 12, Tuesday 30 December 2003
It's pretty peaceful at night here sometimes: the lights are dimmed, and I just sit next to Sophie and hold her hand and often just doze off myself. Just the fact of being there with her means a hell of a lot. I feel as though my responsibility as a father and a husband is being done, and I really try hard to fulfil that role. When I see Sophie asleep, it makes me feel pretty content.

Letter to Sophie, Day 13, Wednesday 31 December 2003
You are in for your second graft and we pray and pray you come through this operation.

You are very good at breathing to relax and helped me today with your physio exercises. Everyone was very proud.

We have more messages of love and support for you from so many people it warms my heart, which often breaks at the sight of you in pain.

Hopefully, you will go in again on Friday to have your head grafted.

We have become desensitised to the pain we see in others in order to focus on you. I will never ever lose compassion, but the tragedy on the ICU can be overwhelming – as is the support from the families of the critically ill and the general public.

We have lost our dreams for our future life and now face the reality of our path together for your care and, hopefully, your inspirational life. I can see this becoming my life's work and relish the challenge of testing all boundaries because you have shown your unbelievable strength.

a bubble of pain

You have taught me courage and how to face my fears, and to have faith and trust because that is what will pull us all through. I love you.

Letter to Sophie, Day 14, Thursday 1 January 2004
Darling girl, you are so sleepy today. You are doing your exercises today so well. You look sad sometimes and it breaks my heart to see you anxious.

We read you stories, tell you how much we love you and give you big hugs full of white light – that is your special hug while you are in hospital as we can't hold you.

Letter to Sophie, Day 15, Friday 2 January 2004
Today, you have your scalp grafted. They may need to grind your skull so that the graft can take because you were burnt deeply on the right side.

You are my brave, courageous princess. I'm so pleased I have had the chance to read stories to you, say prayers with you, sing songs to you, hold your hand – and for you to know I'm holding your hand.

Mitchell has drawn a picture, which is beside your bed, and you look at it through the night when you wake. You watched a video this morning – *Bananas in Pyjamas*. But you're sad because you know you are going to surgery. You left to go to the theatre holding Lilly's hand [Molly Wood's sister].

Ron's journal, Day 15, Friday 2 January 2004
Carolyn and I were very upset today. Everything that's been going on is just weighing heavily on our hearts and our minds. I'm finding it very hard to deal with things at the moment. With

all the lack of sleep and all of the events happening, I seem to be crying a lot. I've asked to see a social worker to talk about that.

Letter to Sophie, Day 16, Saturday 3 January 2004
Today, the ventilator was removed and you are breathing through a tube – we are so proud and feel it is a real milestone. I was able to lie beside you and put my arm around you – it was a privilege, my brave little girl.

You now have a central line [in your chest], and I pray daily that you don't get any infections from it. You are helping the nurses by coughing really well [this helps to clear mucus from the lungs].

Your fight is so hard – a race against time, and the pain and anguish are ever present. Your courage gives me courage to face each day and to offer you all the love and energy I have to help you get strong. The PICU ward is a sad, sad place – the doctors and nurses are unbelievable, given what they face daily. But I will never get bitter; I will retain my compassion, my faith in a higher power, and draw strength from my family and friends.

Catherine has just been with you for twenty-four hours and she sure does keep the nurses on their toes! We appreciate her being here for you so very much.

Today, with Molly, we were labelled the gold-star room!

Letter to Sophie, Day 17, Sunday 4 January 2004
Catherine and John have just been with you and made you laugh!

You have tried to blow bubbles with physio [which also helps to clear the lungs]. You have watched a *Bananas in Pyjamas* video. Mitchell has given you six big kisses, blown onto your nose, chin, forehead, cheeks and lips. Because you are breathing so well, we have been told you can move to the surgical ward as soon as space is available. It's scary, particularly as we were told you would be in ICU for three to four months. We want the best care for you but ward life means we can take more control with your healing, dressings, etc.

Daddy has told me you threw your first tantrum – you wanted more water, which they had fed you in a syringe. You had some licks of lollipop. Your temperature is high and your poo has messed up the bandages – there is always a risk of infection.

Ron's journal, Day 17, Sunday 4 January 2004
Today was the first time that Carolyn was able to have Sophie on her lap. She was just lying there like a mummy, all bandaged up, just her eyes looking around, probably not knowing what was going on. But it was so beautiful to see Sophie on her lap because it may not have ever happened again. You talk about handling someone with kid gloves – even though she's still pretty well morphined out, it was such a delicate procedure to lift her up and to lie her on Carolyn. I think she was with Carolyn for around one and a half hours. We took some photos and it was just a remarkable time – God blessed us to be able to do that – for us and for Sophie.

Over the time we've been here, a lot of our friends have been coming to the waiting room in Intensive Care. At times, we've had fifteen people or so coming to visit. It has got to the point where we've had so much noise being made by our friends that we've had some of the nurses coming out from Intensive Care asking us to be a bit quieter. It's really difficult, because there are so many people who are supporting us. I must admit we've got a few friends who are quite loud, though, so we are continually trying to keep voices down and move to other areas of the hospital to see them. At some stages, it has been pretty chaotic.

Letter to Sophie, Day 18, Monday 5 January 2004

You want 'more ice now!'. This morning, Tricia, your nurse, gave you a big cup of orange juice, which seemed to satisfy. You slept well today, making up for yesterday – a day full of catnaps till 3 am, when they gave you more sedative. You are vocalising well and able to tell the nurses where you hurt. You are blowing bubbles well and coughing well, and for that you got a chocolate milkshake.

I met with the social worker, Sandra Spalding, to get coping techniques for a two-year-old's frustrations at not being able to do what you would like to do.

Unfortunately, Damian confirmed today they were not able to save your right ear at all. But he thought the thumb on your left hand was improving – they may be able to leave the tip.

Tricia said she has never seen anyone do as well in recovery from such severe wounds. You named your baby doll Tricia today.

chapter two
making rainbows

Three weeks in, the initial shock subsides. But now the marathon begins in earnest – the ongoing rounds of operations to graft Sophie's skin, the repeated battles with infection. It is both a marathon and a sprint: in the short term, the doctors are racing against time to get Sophie's skin grafted before infection or organ failure takes hold. Carolyn and Ron marshal their resources: meditation, energy, support, research.

Fittingly, the first big fund-raiser for Sophie and Molly is The Journey: a walk from the Roundhouse to Manly Wharf, from where about three hundred kayaks and surf skis will set off on a thirty-five-kilometre course to Parramatta Stadium, before a smaller group will set out on foot for the Children's Hospital. It has been organised by former Olympic swimming gold medallist Mark Tonelli and ex-Ironman champion Craig Riddington, both friends of the Delezio family, to raise $100,000 for Sophie and Molly and their families. The initial focus of fund-raising is on raising money to support the families with the medical expenses associated with the girls' care.

Later, Ron and Carolyn set up the Day of Difference Foundation to raise funds for hospital equipment and burns research, provide support for children and their families on their journey from emergency to recovery, and advocate for child safety and acceptance of children who are different.

Sophie's hospital support team extends well beyond the doctors and nurses who care for her each day. Also working on her care and recovery are physiotherapists, a social worker, occupational therapists, pain-management specialists, clown doctors – even her own ward granny, a volunteer specially assigned to sit with her and keep her company while Ron and Carolyn meet with doctors or snatch a precious hour of rest.

Letter to Sophie, Day 19, Tuesday 6 January 2004
I cried a lot today.

You came through another operation for 'maintenance'. You have lost some grafts on your left arm. Your lines were blocking. You were sick and Catherine had to clean you up; she made sure you were really comfortable and sleeping peacefully. Staffing issues!

Ron's journal, Day 19, Tuesday 6 January 2004
Sophie had a pretty calm night except she was complaining about sore knees. I wish it were my knees that were sore instead of hers.

Letter to Sophie, Day 20, Wednesday 7 January 2004
Today was a blue day for me; I struggled with my energy levels. Little things got me down and you developed the habit of saying 'no, don't want to' about everything. The team have been called in to think up 'how to entertain' strategies.

A massive fund-raiser is being organised: The Journey, a paddle and walk from the Roundhouse to the hospital. A cocktail auction night is being held on Sunday 18 January.

I've cried a lot for you today.

Letter to Sophie, Day 21, Thursday 8 January 2004
Well, Sophie, it's clear you just don't like being where you are right now. I made the mistake of saying to Mitchell, 'Go to the shops with Dad and get some chips.' You said, 'I want go Daddy shops,' and got very upset. In fact, you are still upset. Most days, we get smiles and calm. Grandma reads stories, Daddy blows bubbles and makes jokes, Grandpa plays with all your teddies and Catherine makes you smile. I just hold your hand.

I'm totally exhausted and emotionally drained. But I am still in awe of your courage and resilience.

Letter to Sophie, Day 22, Friday 9 January 2004
A big op today – more grafts. You will come back with tubes. The beeper goes and my legs turn to lead; I take shallow breaths and dread the doctors' meeting.

All went well with the grafts but the ever-present race against time is a real issue. I thank God for each day and dare to dream of the future, and then become fearful for what that may hold.

You coughed so much your tubes came out your mouth. They will now feed you directly into your stomach and see how you go.

Indi [another Westmead patient] passed today.

Letter to Sophie, Day 23, Saturday 10 January 2004
Let's concentrate on what you can do:
– blink
– breathe
– smile
– listen to music
– sleep
– watch TV and video
– talk when your tubes are out
– rest to help your body get better
– count numbers
– learn colours.
I've been reading books on meditation.

Your tubes were taken out today and you are much happier. Lilly [Wood] made you laugh with the lion talking on the phone.

Kathryn, one of your nurses, came to visit you tonight, just to check on your progress. Gemma is your nurse and she is lovely too. You have a team who care about you a lot in hospital, and we are so grateful for that.

Letter to Sophie, Day 24, Sunday 11 January 2004
We had more smiles and happy faces from you today than we have had before. Grandpa Allan [Martin] played with all your teddy bears and you laughed. He is going back to New Zealand for ten days to pack up their house. [Carolyn's parents moved to Sydney to be closer to Sophie and her family.]

Your antibiotics were stopped today – and then restarted as your temps raced to forty-plus. We call them the 'big guns'. You were sick twice after your chocolate milkshake – only two sips each time – so the dietician is being called in to advise. Pain management will be called in to discuss the pain in your right ear and nerve endings.

I felt you were more peaceful today.

Mitchell left to go home today and said he was going to the beach. You said you didn't want Mitchell to go. Then, 'I want to go to beach too.' Your entertainment will be our biggest challenge.

More messages of support arrive daily and the prayers are worldwide. The community spirit that surrounds both you and Molly is truly inspiring; you have touched so many hearts.

Ron and Carolyn have friends and family in many countries across the globe, but the international prayer chain gains its own life through word of mouth and spreads from country to country.

International Prayer Chain
   Australia
   Canada
   Denmark
   East Africa
   England
   France
   Germany
   Ireland
   Italy
   Korea
   Malaysia
   Malta
   New Zealand
   Singapore
   South Africa
   South America (Mexico, Colombia, Brazil)
   Thailand
   USA (Wisconsin, California, Illinois, Oregon)

Ron's journal, Day 24, Sunday 11 January 2004
It's been a pretty awful day today, with Sophie having high temperatures, above thirty-nine most of the day. There's only one reason for temperatures, and that's infection; she's already got around nine different antibiotics going through her body at the moment.

Letter to Sophie, Day 25, Monday 12 January 2004
Today, you vomited into my hands and had many bouts of diarrhoea – temps as high as 39.9. You only slept for one and a half hours. Your back was itchy like 'mozzy bites', your 'feet' hurt and your shoulder was sore.

The play therapist read you stories and you were quiet and settled. Sandra came to visit and she said she would read you some stories too. She will also work on getting you a ward granny – a volunteer who will be specially assigned to sit with you.

You were pretty miserable today and you just wanted us to be near you. All I wanted to do was hold you and rock you and sing to you, and it broke my heart not to be able to do it for you. I long to hold you in my arms.

But you make it well and truly known when the doctors and nurses are near that you are not happy – loudly exclaiming 'don't touch me!'.

We moved your little body so much today and you bravely blew bubbles [imaginary ones – a pain-management technique]: pink, purple, green and blue with stripes, spots, zigzags and swirls of a variety of colours. We bounce them along clouds, which rain down on grass and grow flowers of many colours – you do it so well, my darling.

Ron's journal, Day 25, Monday 12 January 2004
Sophie is complaining about pain in her foot. The doctors

making rainbows

and nurses had warned us that this could happen – phantom pain in areas that aren't there any more. They've got drugs that they give kids for that and Sophie was given the drugs accordingly.

Every time that Sophie comes up with a new pain, it is important for us to relay that to the nurse, for us to say that she has a pain here or a pain there. We've bought these colourful Wiggles Band-Aids and every time Sophie has a pain we put the Band-Aid where she says the pain is, on the outside of her dressings, so the nurse would see Wiggles Band-Aids on all different parts of the body, showing where the pains are.

Letter to Sophie, Day 26, Tuesday 13 January 2004
A more settled day for everyone. You had good sleeps, smiles and stories; you did puzzles with me and pressed toys. You asked for Lilly Wood to come and play – she loves to use the princess phone. We recommenced your feeds slowly. You asked for chocolate milk and honey toast. Jessica [a friend from the Roundhouse] came and shared an ice-cream cake for her second birthday and you loved the chocolate ice cream best. You asked for Rice Bubbles. I said you could have them for breakfast.

You did more puzzles with me today, read books, played the tambourine with your two fingers. You held your squeezy ball and pressed the Pooh Bear book.

Your feeds recommenced; the second tube is now in your tummy and the vomiting seems to have stopped. You have a rectal tube that reduces any direct contact with poo on your skin – we do not want any more infection. Peter Hayward said he might change your dressings and look at your donor sites on Friday before your big graft Thursday week. So we wait . . . and wait . . .

Ron's journal, Day 26, Tuesday 13 January 2004
Sophie's temperatures continue. I just feel so helpless at the moment, absolutely helpless. Thank God we can go back and have dinner with the Woods tonight; Scott's planning a curry, so I'm looking forward to that – just getting away from the whole thing for an hour or so at least. Then back into it.

Letter to Sophie, Day 27, Wednesday 14 January 2004
I lay by your side tonight and you cried and cried. Your heart rate is up and so is your temperature. You have a pain in your left knee. More sedatives were given to calm you and help you sleep. I was lucky enough to hold you totally. This meant lifting you on pillows while I sat propped up by pillows too.

You had the clown doctors come and see you; they sang you songs and blew bubbles. They made you a pink poodle out of balloons. Mitchell came today and you showed him how you pressed buttons.

You were given the most beautiful quilt today from Quilts for Keeps – it's your own special blanket for your bed. The pattern is called Superstars; I liked it because that's what everyone calls you.

Father Paul and Sister Bridget came and blessed you and me today. They have lent us the most beautiful cross, made from timber taken from Mary MacKillop's school, and I will use it daily to say prayers for you.

John Delezio came and fed you Rice Bubbles and told us funny stories of his paddling training for The Journey, which is being held for you and Molly on Sunday.

Letter to Sophie, Day 28, Thursday 15 January 2004
Sophie, you had an unsettled night and an 'I sad' morning. After

making rainbows

41

a little sleep, you were happier, especially when Mitchell and Lilly Wood came to play. The play therapist, Lisa, came with more toys with buttons to press and you were very proud to show how you could make all the sounds.

You asked me to take you to the toilet – 'you take me' – and said 'I go now' when you wanted to get out of bed. It's hard when you are sad because no amount of distractions will help change your mood. You seem to just need a good sleep.

You have Wiggles Band-Aids all over but they seem to help with the pain. You have bangles on your arm and look just beautiful.

You blew beautiful bubbles with spots and zigzags and a variety of colours. Big soft bubbles bouncing up to the clouds, filling them with water to grow grass and colourful flowers. You amaze everyone with your bravery and we continue to get messages, presents and prayers. The parents and grandparents of other very sick children are also amazingly compassionate.

Ron's journal, Day 28, Thursday 15 January 2004
Sophie has been crying a lot; she even told us that she is very sad, and that absolutely broke our hearts. We had to go and see the social worker to have a look at that, just to make sure we were covering all angles in terms of Sophie getting out of this whole mess. It's not just a physical thing, it's a psychological thing that we're battling now.

Poor little thing, she's had to have some of her bandages redone because she had done big poos. We had to put Jelonet dressing on, so she is upset and distressed. Every time someone needs to go near her or touch her, Sophie gets very upset. She doesn't want anyone to touch her; I don't really blame her, but we need to do what we have to do.

Letter to Sophie, Day 29, Friday 16 January 2004
You said to me, 'A beach ball hurt me,' after waking this morning. You have your big op today. Your cultured skin is coming from Concord; we have a theatre booked for the whole day just for you and an air bed at the ready. [The 'air loss mattress' offers extra stability without pressing on healing burns – it is put on top of the regular hospital bed.]

The Concord team arrived: Dr Peter Maitz, who developed your cultured skin, and the nurse who looked after it. It was split-second timing. Peter Hayward said he had never had so many people in theatre with him before. Damian attended, although he had officially left on Monday.

You came out prone [face down] with a special jacket on, lying on the air bed; you have your tubes in your nose again. They are hoping to extubate you tomorrow.

Peter said we kicked goals today. You are eighty-five per cent burnt and he has covered half of you in grafts with your own skin or the one metre of cultured skin that was grown. You have spray-on skin [another form of cultured skin] growing in Western Australia.

Ron's journal, Day 29, Friday 16 January 2004
I miss Mitchell a lot when he's not here. Miss being at home, miss everything being normal. We know we'll never see that again, though I suppose it's only early days.

Today was a big day – the cultured skin was brought from Concord to graft onto Sophie's back. We were waiting outside theatre for the skin to arrive and all of a sudden the doctors arrived, the nurses, the scientists from Concord Skin Culture Laboratory, bringing the skin with them in an ordinary esky! It's amazing – all this technology and they still just put it in an esky to keep it cool.

Letter to Sophie, Day 30, Saturday 17 January 2004
It's shades of the first week – you are frustrated at not being able to talk, so your blood pressure races. We do physio exercises three times a day. You are being weaned off morphine. Your nose runs and you dribble all the time; I wipe it clean for you. Your eyes are swollen because of all the fluid pressure.

I find it difficult to comfort you because I reminisce about times gone by, particularly your first week in hospital. So short, regular times are best for me to assist you. Daddy and I take it in turns. We were advised that it is often one step back to take the next step forward, and that's a very real picture for us. It breaks my heart to see you like this.

Therese came and harmonised you again today; she said your energy field is much firmer.

Letter to Sophie, Day 31, Sunday 18 January 2004
The Journey 2004 began with thousands walking from the Roundhouse to Manly; two hundred paddlers were cheered off from Manly Beach heading to Parramatta; and a final group walked to Westmead, with firefighters at every stop. The cocktail party was originally ticketed for three hundred; they sold three hundred and seventy-eight, and Diesel and INXS were playing. Linda took loads of photos so we can see just how many people are supporting you.

Mid-afternoon, the walkers entered the hospital grounds. More T-shirts were sold – there were red 'Journey' hats everywhere. Scott Wood made a speech with Craig Riddington and Mark Tonelli. Ron went to the cocktail party and made a speech on your behalf. Lexus had a car and driver available for us the whole day, taking family here and there.

You were extubated today and as soon as you could talk

wanted 'more ice now'. You had an unsettled night; Trish gave you something to 'sleep better'.

Dad stayed with you till 1.30 am reading you stories and feeding you ice. Grandma Joy [Martin] spent time with you and so did Catherine.

Ron's journal, Day 31, Sunday 18 January 2004
The big day of the paddle in Manly. It started at the Roundhouse; it was an absolutely surreal experience, going back to the place where this nightmare all started. We were met down there by the mayor and lots of friends and thousands of people. We walked from there down to Manly Wharf and there were people with Sophie T-shirts and Sophie caps on everywhere, doing the fund-raiser and paddling from there to Parramatta. What a fantastic experience: I was on a boat most of the way and John was paddling with a mate; Scott paddled from a certain point as well and I met them both just before Parramatta and paddled the rest of the way with them.

Letter to Sophie, Day 32, Monday 19 January 2004
What a sad day you had – all you could do was say 'I sad'. Your bottom lip trembles and I ache to hold you in my arms. You have to go to surgery again today, which I am so scared about. You have an infection, *Pseudomonas*, which for you is critical; we all hope it hasn't affected the skin on your back.

I cried next to your bed because I saw the anguish on your face whenever the doctors' teams came by. You went to surgery mid-afternoon and came out about 6.30 pm. Each operation you have is about three hours long, because it takes that long just to change your dressings.

Great news: your right arm was severely infected but your back had only a couple of small spots, which they think they caught in time. You arrived back prone, intubated and heavily sedated, so you have a settled night.

Ron's journal, Day 32, Monday 19 January 2004
I noticed early this morning that Sophie's dressings on her back and bottom and neck look pretty green, and there were no green areas when they last turned her at nine o'clock the night before. This happens really fast. Suddenly, bang! You've got a major infection.

Letter to Sophie, Day 33, Tuesday 20 January 2004
The public support for you is truly inspirational, boosting my spirits to face another day.

It's much easier to see you sedated, as you rest well and don't get as distressed. You've had two incidents that have left you intubated; your stats dropped. I have not been a hundred per cent, so Mum came and sat with you while I had an hour's rest in the middle of the day – the first in five weeks.

Your tubes came out and you asked for water, chocolate and yoghurt. You said, 'I'm scared – I'm sad.' I'm holding your hand and will never ever let it go. Your neurological pain has kicked in again. You want to hold blankie but can't feel it in your hand.

They have to make up your feeds to ensure you have a minimum intake over the course of each week, since you end up having to fast for days because of all your procedures.

Letter to Sophie, Day 34, Wednesday 21 January 2004
You wake early and watch videos. This morning, from 9.30, you were saying, 'I want Mummy, I want Daddy, I'm scared, I'm sad,' and you were being very demanding.

You wanted water and you wanted it now. You didn't want ice; you wanted chocolate milk and a chocolate doughnut. You wanted orange juice; you didn't want books or games, just videos and music. You said at lunchtime you wanted to sleep and we put music on but you didn't sleep – you haven't slept all day. I said it's important to sleep so your body can get better but you just don't seem to rest easy during the days.

I went home to pick up Mitchell and came straight back; it's now 7.15 pm and you have only just settled. It worries me you are not getting more rest and I will be discussing it with the team of doctors tonight and again tomorrow. You will be operated on again tomorrow – a dressing change and a new rectal tube. You will be fasted from 4 am for a 10 am start and we face the same old issue of your diet yet again. You keep saying, 'Help me, Mummy. Help me, Mummy.'

Ron's journal, Day 34, Wednesday 21 January 2004
It's funny how things turn around: after having to get ice for Sophie so many times, she's now down to 35.5 and too cold. So blankets all over her, the overhead heating on, trying to heat her up again.

Letter to Sophie, Day 35, Thursday 22 January 2004
What an exciting day! You went to surgery for a dressing change at 11 am. Beforehand, you were very sleepy, doing a catch-up after not sleeping for the past two days. Peter Hayward came out of theatre into the PICU waiting room saying, 'Where are the Delezios?' Reception had us on the phone and he was saying, 'It's a miracle, it's a miracle.' Peter Maitz, Peter Hayward and [doctor] Andrew Williams were all very pleased with how well your cultured skin had taken. This is the first time Concord has sent cultured skin off-site and it worked so well on a large area.

'Growing like grass,' says Peter Hayward. It's wonderful news and we have smiles from ear to ear; we are enjoying a positive day. You came back totally sedated with a tube in your mouth; they want you prone for three days. Your eyes are swollen and mucus runs from your nose and mouth, but it's better out than in! Peter says the scales are now tipped your way. Now we dare make plans for the future.

In order for the grafts to take on her back, the largest area of damaged skin, Sophie has to remain face down for long periods of time. She is also sedated so that the grafts will take, which means that she has to be intubated for her breathing.

Letter to Sophie, Day 36, Friday 23 January 2004

Friday was a rest day for us as well as you. It's amazing how relieved we feel when you sleep. We wander in and out of the room not knowing what to do because you are so still – all chemically induced, of course, but the plan is to keep you heavily sedated so that your skin can really take. You are supposed to be prone, sedated and intubated for three days, so we'll see how the plan goes. You are due for a dressing change – your back only – on the weekend. It looks like it will be Sunday at this stage and may be done in the ward – a first. Andrew wants to give you a break from surgery next week so your donor site can heal. We'll see what Peter [Hayward] has to say and what unfolds during the week: each day is different, bringing with it the unexpected. I'm pleased we had a happy ending to a very difficult week; the good times help you get through the tough days and we know there will be many more ahead. You are having a psychological assessment on Tuesday because your beautiful smile isn't around much any more.

Letter to Sophie, Day 37, Saturday 24 January 2004
You sleep a little but not a lot, so again I'm having the same discussions I seem to have with every new nurse – about keeping you sedated and comfortable. We had a big fright at midday when your temperature spiked at forty as your dressings came off. I had not seen your back exposed before. The air conditioning was lowered and a fan was brought in; you were packed in ice and given ibuprofen and paracetamol. Ron stood and fanned you while they tracked a fan down – all too scarce in a PICU ward.

Your BMP reading came down over the hour and you will continue to be gently fanned to keep you stable. They are running blood cultures to see what the infection is.

You are so thirsty; you call out for water all the time. Unfortunately, all you can have is a few drops on a pink sponge. If I am with you, you get distressed at me not giving you more water, which just distresses me more. You have devised a way of showing your displeasure – you move your bottom up into the air and down. It's just as if you were stomping your feet.

Letter to Sophie, Day 38, Sunday 25 January 2004
You had your dressings changed today – just your back. Peter Hayward, Andrew, Kathryn and Irene were in attendance. Everyone was very happy with your back. You were able to lie on your back on the air bed after your dressing change – it must be more comfortable.

You seem to have had a very peaceful day – then I remembered that you were given extra morphine twice this afternoon in anticipation of having your central line changed and being extubated. Your dressings were changed in your room this morning because it was just a matter of unwrapping the special jacket you wear and replacing it. You haven't had your dressings changed in PICU since the first week, when you were too sick to have them done anywhere else. Sister Bridget came to see you today and Petrea King [Quest for Life founder] came to see us too, giving us tips on making rainbows [spiritual visualisation]. She is a wonderful lady who gave me some very useful tools.

Ron's journal, Day 38, Sunday 25 January 2004
Carolyn and I had the night at home with Mitchell. It was good to come in and see Sophie – the nurses said things went pretty well last night. I just feel so guilty leaving the hospital, leaving Sophie there. But you've got to follow your heart and we know that we've got to spend that one night with Mitchell at home, to make sure he still knows we're there for him, that we love him and we care.

Letter to Sophie, Day 39, Monday 26 January 2004
You have had a more awake day and did some puzzles. Tricia read stories and we played music. Daddy had you laughing and playing with bubble mix; Mitchell drew you a picture with magic numbers on it. He sat on my knee and you said, 'No Mitchell on Mummy's knee.' Mitchell jumped off and said, 'Okay, Sophie.' Then you said, 'I want sit on Mummy's knee.' I said we would talk to the doctor about it.

Your temperature spiked again today – we had the fan to cool you. We packed you in ice. Your rectal tube leaked again, so it was a matter of a quick bandage/dressing check while you were rolled from side to side. You blew the best imaginary bubbles – big ones, little ones, soft ones and all manner of colours – and bounced them all the way to the purple cloud. You are learning all about rainbows – being wrapped in them and receiving them into your heart. You can send them to whomever you want to. You sent one to me today and I sent one to Daddy.

chapter three
the price of innocence

Six weeks after Sophie's accident, Carolyn starts keeping a private journal. It is the dark underside of her letter to Sophie: raw and emotional, it lays bare the fear, anger and pain she is feeling and her struggle to deal with what has happened to her child.

Around this time, Carolyn makes the decision to give up work in order to devote herself to Sophie's care. She has been in the process of acquiring a rental-management company and was due to sign the final purchase papers on 16 December, the day after Sophie's accident.

Ron and Carolyn also have to deal with the 'business side' of Sophie's accident, negotiating with lawyers as they strive to establish where fault lies. As the law stood at that time, victims of a no-fault accident were not entitled to any compensation through the compulsory green-slip insurance scheme. If they don't receive an insurance payout, Ron and Carolyn are faced with selling their house and everything they have in order to pay for Sophie's care. (After the

Delezio case, the New South Wales government expanded the scope of the scheme's coverage. In the end, the insurance company did make a payout to Sophie's family.)

It is only on Day 45 that the doctors declare Sophie clear of brain injuries. The extreme heat from the car engine under which she was trapped burnt Sophie's head through to the skull, and there was a very real possibility that her brain may have been damaged. Having secured that crucial all-clear, Ron and Carolyn's immediate goal is to get Sophie well enough to leave Intensive Care and move to the hospital's Burns Unit – Clubbe Ward.

Letter to Sophie, Day 40, Tuesday 27 January 2004
Oh, my darling – what a day. You were moved by three nurses to go prone and your central line came out. Dr David [anaesthetist] said the F word and had to put in a new central line for you. Had it not worked, another trip to theatre would have been needed. Good news: he did it, and we left your bedside at 4 am.

You went to theatre for a dressing change and you have the *Pseudomonas* infection again. We may lose some of the cultured skin – I'm so sad and scared; my mind is in a blur. You are to move to a room of your own so they can control the infection better. I think you will enjoy your new room because you are by the nurses' station and you will be able to watch all the activity.

Peter Hayward wants to graft you again on Thursday if we can get theatre time. Andrew will dress your head in the ward tomorrow.

I love you, my courageous warrior spirit.

Carolyn's journal, Day 40, Tuesday 27 January 2004
Day 40 and I feel as shattered as I did that second week. My legs have turned to lead. I am vague and non-responsive. I look dishevelled and it seems an exhausting job to rally a positive spirit. I'm immensely fearful of losing my daughter. I've lost my

appetite, I want to curl up and go to sleep and wake up from the nightmare, but I can't because this is our reality. I have bile in my tummy and the enormity of the situation hits home to me. We walk in a living hell.

Today, I am consumed with fear and it takes me back to those early weeks I just don't want to remember, when each step down the hospital corridor was a physical effort just to get to sit by my daughter's side. The first two or three days, I was unable to walk unassisted; I needed someone on each arm just to get me to the toilet. I remember talking to the chaplain, Jan, and in a very emotional state asking how you stay sane in a place like this if you have to be here long-term – I did not want the bile and anger to be a part of me. We decided on faith, courage, compassion, spirituality and will. From then on, I felt like I was on a mission to beat the odds!

Even today, I speak with Robyn; she has been here four months with Ben, who was paralysed from the neck down, and she says she can't imagine what Ron and I are going through. This has happened since we first arrived here. At the same time, I've met some amazing people and feel more blessed for the experience. It's funny, as I write this a chopper flies overhead and my blood runs cold, yet in a way I feel slightly anaesthetised; maybe this is the brain's way of coping with a critically ill child, reserving something for the days ahead. The fear is enormous at times. Back in the first or second week, I had to have a counsellor come and see me. It was eleven in the evening and I had an all-consuming fear of the dark; it was immediate and I knew I needed help. The nurses asked if it could wait – the answer was NO, so the counsellor had to drive forty-five minutes to get here. I felt better after the meeting and was able to get a few hours' sleep.

The other overwhelming reality is the shattered lives of not just ourselves but also our friends and family. Mitchell displaced; Mum and Dad moving countries to care for him.

I remember my mother saying [after settling in New Zealand] that she would never move countries again. The loss of my business; the reality that I will never again work full-time. I know from discussions with parents of long-term patients and doctors the huge number of ongoing medical requirements – as Peter Hayward put it, 'for years and years and years and years'.

What price do you put on the loss of innocence? The innocence of a precious two-year-old who will be seriously disabled for the rest of her life.

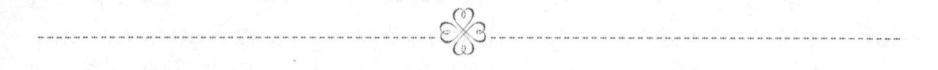

Letter to Sophie, Day 41, Wednesday 28 January 2004
A calmer day for all concerned. You have another infection and are on more IV fluids to supplement your fluid loss. You met Lyn South, your ward granny, today. Geata, Amanda and Laura visited from the Roundhouse, but you were mostly asleep – although you have taken to squeezing your eyes shut when you don't want to see something, particularly doctors and nurses.

Your head was dressed in your room today and Andrew is very happy with how it looks. You are scheduled for theatre tomorrow and they hope to graft your leg. We had a psych team assess you today and they are working on the possibility of antidepressants, since your mood swings prevent you from sleeping at night. They will be doing a lot of research into what may be appropriate and will present us with a research paper tomorrow for consideration. You have had Louise [Jennings] on tonight and Tricia today – a great team. You are sleeping, giving your Tricia doll a cuddle with your arm over her. You have your lullaby music on to help you settle and a few chemicals to keep you sedated and calm.

Ron's journal, Day 41, Wednesday 28 January 2004
Sophie's temperature up to 39.1. We've made so many visits to the ice-making machine it's not funny. Carolyn and I said last

night that when we leave this place, we're going to put an ice machine in ICU so other parents don't have to go all the way to the other ward, which is absolutely ridiculous. If a child needs ice in ICU, they're in a serious condition.

It looks like Sophie is going to theatre again tomorrow afternoon. She's in a sad mood today, needs a lot of attention and reassurance that everything's going to be all right, that we're with her and we'll get through together.

Letter to Sophie, Day 42, Thursday 29 January 2004
Today, you have had another graft on your left leg and arm. We are so proud of you: you came back without a tube, breathing on your own – they put the mask near your face and you said, 'I don't need it.' You were sad and grumpy all day; you want water and ice and can't have it because you throw it up. We need to do more IV fluids to stop you getting so dry.

We all take turns to read you stories, have you listen to music, watch videos and make up stories about us going shopping – creative visualisation to take you away from your hospital room. It's very hands on, about an hour each for ward granny Lyn, Dad, Grandma and me. Jude [friend] arrived from New Zealand with a lot of research on burns and children, and she has even been in touch with Middlemore Hospital Burns Unit [in New Zealand]. It's wonderful having friends on the research team, as our time is taken up each day with caring for you and Mitchell.

Carolyn's journal, Day 42, Thursday 29 January 2004
Sophie is on the emergency list for surgery, so we pray she gets a theatre time. X-rays because of pain when the bowel washout occurs raise her levels of anxiety and mine. I have a constant gnawing in my tummy, part of my fear/anxiety level. I have to

the price of innocence

take deep breaths. This was an issue as soon as the accident happened. On the drive to Westmead, Linda was constantly telling me to be strong and breathe. I carried a paper bag so I could breathe my own oxygen for four days after the accident, after my stay in Westmead Emergency when they thought I was having a stroke.

Ron's journal, Day 42, Thursday 29 January 2004
Had Mitch in today at Sophie's bedside. It was a bit distressing for Mitch that Sophie was really unsettled; it's very unsettling for us, too, to see Sophie that way. I had a bit of a chat to the nurse about giving her a Medazolan infusion. I just don't want to see her in pain; I don't want Mitchell to see her in pain either.

Letter to Sophie, Day 43, Friday 30 January 2004
A settled day – temps of up to 38.8 and lots of vomiting in the morning, but Medazolan seems to be working well to settle you. You are complaining of being sore on your belly button – this could be because you were 'cropped' [your skin harvested] as it's your donor site. You have had spray-on cells put on that site so it heals faster. Peter and Andrew plan to schedule an operation each week to complete your grafts: your right leg, your head, then your two arms. Because you will be able to go onto your back next week after about ten days on your tummy, you may lose some of the back graft. Your morphine level has been put back up to a hundred and this seems to keep you calmer when all your procedures are over. Your feeds are continually on catch-up but Pru [PICU dietician] is pleased with how this has gone; in the last week, you have needed a lot of protein to help heal your grafts and donor site. You are a little sad again this evening and cry but you can't say why, and you vomited again.

Carolyn's journal, Day 43, Friday 30 January 2004
I feel so guilty today because I have had so little time to spend with Mitchell. You can see his emotions change as he becomes more demanding and unsettled. He says, 'I'm scared,' when going to bed and, 'Don't leave me, Mummy,' and it breaks your heart. It's demanding in one sense but totally understandable. The time with Sophie is just as demanding but on a completely different level. Very intense in terms of her care and her entertainment, and a constant battle to get her to sleep so she can have a reasonable amount of rest in terms of her moods. And then you realise you haven't set foot outside the hospital, just in the lifts or up and down a ramp for a little light relief. I'm lucky if I get to make one phone call per day in response to the multiple work, domestic and personal calls. At times, it seems overwhelming even to get the washing done. And everyone is still doing so much for us. Our friends/family have been amazing and without them this road would be too much to bear.

Letter to Sophie, Day 44, Saturday 31 January 2004
Today, I arrive at your bedside and your central line has come out again. I feel panicked but doctors reassure me that morphine is passed through your transpyloric line. Your antibiotics are stopped. You will go to theatre again tomorrow for a new central line and dressing change. Your morphine is increased to ten times the normal dose due to the slower absorption rate. Your temps are 38.2–38.9. Mandy has bought a fan, which the electrical bio-med team will check on Monday [for any problems with wiring, etc. that could affect the hospital's electricity], then we can start using it. We can donate it to PICU afterwards, as they don't have one!

You are so beautiful. Dad took a video of you today eating your first iceblock! It was lemonade. You wanted to hold it yourself and got upset because you can't bend your arm. So we fed you with a spoon from your special Sophie cup.

Ron's journal, Day 44, Saturday 31 January 2004
Came to Sophie's room to find her central line had been pulled out again. Had a meeting with one of the doctors, who explained to me that it had dropped out. I explained back to him that they don't just drop out by themselves and that it was accidentally pulled out. The doctor said that they were giving Sophie her morphine through her transpyloric line, in doses that put Sophie to sleep quite well. Andy came in and said that they will enter a new Hickman line (central line) during the dressing change in theatre tomorrow.

Letter to Sophie, Day 45, Sunday 1 February 2004
You are first up in theatre for your new central line and dressing change but get pushed back. It is a three-hour wait but the news is good: your grafts are looking good. I'm so relieved that your donor site is healing well, because you have been saying that your belly button was sore for the last two days. The fact that your donor site has recovered so well and that your grafts are healing so well means we will only have to have two more major operations: your right leg and your head. Peter Hayward said there will be many more small grafts. He also said today that he feels confident that we won't lose you due to your brain injuries, which was great news. You now have about thirty per cent of your injuries left to graft. You came back from theatre extubated and on your back, which we think is fantastic considering that you had X-rays this morning for a chest infection. You still have a staph [*Staphylococcus*] infection and we are waiting for the results of tests for other infections.

Ron's journal, Day 45, Sunday 1 February 2004
It doesn't matter how many times I go to theatre with Sophie, I still end up falling apart and crying (though not in front of her). Sophie came back from theatre and Peter Hayward and Andy were very happy with her skin grafts. Peter said that Sophie has around thirty per cent of her body still to cover and he believes that she is now not threatened by the damage to her skin. He believes the only threat could be if her kidneys or other organs failed. He said that he is quite comfortable for Sophie to go to the Burns Unit if ICU says it's okay. Barry (PICU doctor) said maybe in a couple of days. Sophie slept well and woke telling me she doesn't love me. I know how frustrated she is and accept how much anger and confusion is bottled up inside of her.

Letter to Sophie, Day 46, Monday 2 February 2004
When we arrived at your bed today, you had been sick. You had blown out another rectal tube, so you had to have your dressings changed. Your temp is 39.8, so we packed you in ice, got your fan going, helped make your bed with new sheets and blueys [disposable bed pads], told you stories while all this was happening – about the ginger cat and friends playing tennis – held your hand, counted and did big breaths to help ease the trauma of you being moved. You insist on ice, water and 'now'. We are having to remind you of your manners.

But you are so beautiful; it's lovely to see you on your back. You try so hard to help with physio exercises and with dressing changes, moving your legs and arms. I climb in at your request to lie next to you in bed. I did this again this evening around midnight so you could sleep. My sweet baby girl.

We visit the Burns ward because it looks like you will be moved tomorrow. You will have your own room – you will be isolated because of the staph virus you have.

Carolyn's journal, Day 46, Monday 2 February 2004
We walk into Sophie's room not knowing what to expect. Ron thinks the hardest part is that first entry. She had been sick, blown out her rectal tube and had a temp of 39.8. Her vomit ran down one side of her dressing, her poo was over her legs and it's a logistical exercise getting her dressed and tidied. We want Lisa [one of the Intensive Care doctors] to assure us Sophie's chest infection is okay. We want more info on her other infections: staph, *Pseudomonas* and any others that might have crept up.

Peter is keen to see Sophie in the Burns ward. He has called the ward pretty well all day. Wants her there for her mental health. He also said the central line will be an ongoing issue and he has been right, as we have lost two this week.

Jude has done a heap of research on burns survivors for us. The psych team have given us some info on medications; we are unsure what to do! To see if she needs more meds, we will monitor her behaviour over the next three days. Ron said he felt numb when Peter and Andrew met with us post-op yesterday. It's hard to get excited about any good news because her situation changes daily. It is emotionally draining. I can't focus on work, paying bills – even making my one phone call a day is an effort to keep up with.

Ron's journal, Day 46, Monday 2 February 2004
Sophie was watching the end of *Ice Age* when we arrived. She spoke to Mitchell on the phone. She seemed very quiet and sad. Brad (nurse) said Sophie will be going to the Burns Unit tomorrow and that he would take us around for a look this afternoon. Caro attended the unit meeting downstairs while I stayed with Sophie. Sophie is to have a head dressing this afternoon. Bit of a vomit. David (nurse) and I helped to clean her up, cutting away some of the contaminated dressing. It hurts her a lot when we turn her around for this clean-up. It hurts me to see Sophie in any pain at all. Found Sophie looking

down at her legs in a sort of trance. I hoped she wouldn't ask any questions. Asked her to tell me what's on the video to distract her attention. I don't know how I am going to handle telling Sophie about her legs.

Scared about Sophie going to the Burns Unit tomorrow. She will go from 24/7 one-on-one care to a ward where no one will be in her room except for nurse rounds. I think either Caro or I will be spending a lot more time with Sophie, especially at night. Probably we will take turns sleeping with her.

Had a discussion with Trudy [friend] about the extent of fund-raising. Went to check out the Burns ward with Caro and Joy. A bit scary, but we know it's got to the next step on Sophie's journey to get out of here. I went back to the unit around 10.30 pm; Caro ended up in bed with Sophie until 1 am before joining me. Another day that we can leave behind us; another day that we don't have to worry about again.

Letter to Sophie, Day 47, Tuesday 3 February 2004
You ask for water and ice at 8.30 am. You throw up and your rectal tube has leaked, so we need to change your dressings. Your temp overnight got to 39.8. You may need to go to theatre; the doctors are assessing the central line they put in on Sunday – it's too close to your heart. You are fasted anticipating their decision. They decide Wednesday is the day, so you can recommence taking ice and water to quench your thirst. Your temperature settles and, after some chloral hydrate, you sleep finally, after twelve hours.

You tell me you are 'not happy' as we try to space the fluid intake so you don't vomit. I've had a visit from Katy, Olivia's mum [Olivia was another of the children at the Roundhouse on that day], which is lovely; everyone offers help. John from Stella Maris College visited too, with a teddy and a balloon for you.

He is a religious teacher and wants to do something to help you and Molly get well. I said, 'Just pray.'

Carolyn's journal, Day 47, Tuesday 3 February 2004
I feel shattered. It's 4.45 pm and I just want to sleep. My mind is just not sharp: I can only just hold a conversation without getting confused, losing the storyline or thinking of other things. Today, we should have been in the Burns Unit. But instead (and we should know better), we are facing another theatre trip. I had just hoped Sophie could have a break so we could re-establish all her routines that we had tried to establish with diet, physio, play, sleep. Sophie was being fasted and she was desperate for water. Fortunately, Trish, her night nurse, had given her an extra bag of fluid because of her thirst. I broke down when I went to change her ice packs because of her overnight 39.8 temp and she lay with her mouth wide open crying. No parent should ever see their child so desperate. David Murrell, the anaesthetic registrar, was furious when he came on rounds because we had been waiting for three hours – no decision had been made. He raced around stirring everyone up to make a decision. They have now put off surgery till tomorrow, so we feed water and iceblocks to Sophie to quench her thirst. Her feeds are recommenced, thank goodness, and catch-up is again played.

Ron's journal, Day 47, Tuesday 3 February 2004
Left early for home to have a meeting with Rebecca Riddington [Craig's wife]. Rebecca will be working for Scott and myself in coordinating donations and events. Rod Smith [solicitor] also mentioned that, as we are starting our own charity, we will need someone to handle it on a full-time basis. Arrived back at the hospital to find out that Sophie was not going to the Burns Unit because the central line that was fitted on Sunday was inserted too far into the heart and was touching the valve. Andy said that the X-ray for ICU showed it going in 16 mm too far; it was

not that serious but needed to be fixed soon. No time has been given yet but Sophie has been placed on the emergency list for Wednesday.

Letter to Sophie, Day 48, Wednesday 4 February 2004
You are fasted from 6 am and go to theatre at 2 pm. You wake up and call for water/ice/straw/special cup and it is continuous. We feed you ice, which you crunch happily. Your tummy is aspirated so all the fluid is removed, otherwise you would vomit. Every time something goes in, it comes out again. This way, you can have fluids till noon. Trish has given you extra fluids and caught up your feeds overnight. You were calling her by name and telling her about your home. Bettina was on today and she is lovely with you. You now have a small bell to ring when you want water. You went to theatre gripping it like nothing else. Your dressings were changed and your Hickman line taken back so it poses no potential harm to your heart. You are now scheduled to go to the Burns Unit tomorrow. Your infections are being tracked; your lungs are okay – only a small weakness remains. You tell me that you can't get your toes out. I said it's okay, the bandages are making you better.

Carolyn's journal, Day 48, Wednesday 4 February 2004
Kam Soon, the anaesthetic doctor, stopped me in the hall and said, 'You need to take time out. You have a marathon ahead of you.' I recalled something of the first week; I got flashbacks about it. An hour later, I want to write it here and can't remember again.

I had a conversation with Mary [friend, business adviser] today. Following her request for approval to move the office, Matthew [not his real name] indicated to her that it was my business anyway. Alarm bells started ringing and I resigned as licensee; I did not want to go through with a business acquisition with someone playing a hard line, given our present circumstances. It made me really angry that when we were in theatre with my daughter I was concerned about Matthew and his reaction to the move of offices. It became clear that I am not in a position to spend the time I need to on running a business and I do not need the extra pressure. Sophie's needs must come first, so my dreams of owning, running and building a business have just been shattered.

Catherine came to theatre with us. Ron, Cath and myself sat there in a row and shed tears for Sophie. I'm sure Cath's tears were for her dad too. My legs have been wobbly today, my tummy agitated and I have no appetite. Soph's grafts are doing well, though she lost some graft on the tops of her legs due to poo.

It's good to hear the good news – it's amazing how tolerant you become of the bad. I wanted to go to Lucas's funeral and couldn't leave because of theatre – it's just too hard to make any plans. Sue, Lucas's mum, was such a strength to me at the beginning. I felt it was the least I could have done and that I have let Sue and Lucas down by not being there. I share their pain.

Ron's journal, Day 48, Wednesday 4 February 2004
Sophie had a good sleep last night and Tricia said that Sophie was talking about our home. The operation to adjust the Broviac line was to be at 12 noon but ended up at 2.30 pm. I am so sick and tired of it – the poor thing fasts almost every second day in preparation for surgery. It's so damn complicated.

Anyway, Sophie came back to her room at 4.15 pm; we spoke to Andy, who said he was extremely happy with the skin grafts. A bit missing here and there, but generally going extremely well. Andy wants us down on the Burns ward asap. Sophie was peaceful when she came back in. Wanted more water again. Sophie always loved her water, so it's even harder for her not to be able to drink that much.

Mitchell came over with Carolyn Reid [friend] and was happy to see us all again. We were told that Sophie and Molly are both going to the Burns ward tomorrow.

Scott and I went to the Burns Unit with his doctor (and head of burns), John [Harvey]. He showed Scott the ward and we sat down and had a brief meeting on tomorrow's move. Sophie will have to be isolated due to her having MRSA – Methicillin-resistant *Staphylococcus aureus* [an antibiotic-resistant form of the staph infection]. Apparently, this is a common infection in children who are in hospital for long periods of time. The unfortunate thing is that MRSA cannot be treated with antibiotics. It will go as her immune system picks up when she is healthier. So Molly and Sophie need to be in separate rooms, at least until Sophie is cleared of the MRSA. Never mind. At least, or at most, we are getting out of ICU after fifty-two days. The change of scenery and quietness are going to help Sophie heal. I am getting more excited all the time about the move.

Spoke to Rod Smith about Caro not taking up the offer to buy Matthew's business. Apparently, Matthew had said to Mary that as far as he is concerned it is Caro's business and that she can on-sell it if she wants. I said to Caro and Rod that she should resign as licensee of Prime Link and tell Matthew a date that Caro and Mary will no longer take part in the business. Well, at last the decision was made by Caro – that she would not buy the company. Caro is officially a full-time mum. A big decision.

Caro advised Rod that Amanda had seen the car crashing in through the wall and that she said the driver's eyes were open as he crashed. This is contrary to what other people said. They all said that he was unconscious at the time of impact, which supports his story. [The driver of the car, Don McNeall, was later found not guilty of negligent driving causing grievous bodily harm, as the magistrate could not rule out the possibility that McNeall had suffered a seizure.]

We had dinner with Scott and Caroline, as we have had for the last fifty-one days.

chapter four
out of Intensive Care

A new phase of the journey commences: Sophie is moved to the Burns Unit. This means less intensive-nursing support; the flipside is that Ron and Carolyn must shoulder more responsibility for Sophie's care. The move spells progress but at the same time it strips the family of the tenuous sense of stability that Intensive Care has come to represent.

Although Sophie's condition is no longer considered critical enough for her to be kept in the PICU unit, sudden high temperatures suggest that an infection from the central line might be taking hold, which in Sophie's condition could be fatal. On Day 52, Carolyn writes, 'I get fearful and panicked that we may still lose Sophie.'

Letter to Sophie, Day 49, Thursday 5 February 2004
Peter Hayward visited you in the Burns Unit and said, 'They said we wouldn't make it.'

We pack up all your belongings and feel the excitement of

a new phase in your care. Dad videos Molly's departure in the morning; yours is scheduled for the afternoon.

We arrive and you have a beautiful pink myrtle tree outside your sunny room. You and Molly share a nurse, for which we are very grateful. One of us will sleep by your bed each night; you have a sofa chair that we will use. I'm with you from 4 pm as Mitchell and Dad go shopping. You sleep at 1 am for an hour, then again at 4 am. It is exhausting: you want water, chicken bones [drumsticks], rice, my dinner, your dinner, ice, etc. You run temperatures, need bowel washouts, turning and medications that constantly disturb any chance of a restful night. I feel the need to write you a program so Ron and I can keep a check on your rehab plan. I will draw up an Excel spreadsheet over the weekend. We eat at 10.30 pm. Routines need to be established.

Ron's journal, Day 49, Thursday 5 February 2004
Sophie had a fairly restless night; they used up all the drugs they had to try to get her to sleep. I followed Scott, Caroline and Molly down to Burns at 11 am and took photos of their move. So much stuff builds up in Sophie's room over time that I needed a trolley to move it all down. Great room. Plenty of sun and a door leading out to a grassed play area with trees, a play centre, slippery dip, etc. Ideal for Mitchell.

Earlier in the morning, I had a meeting with John Harvey, head of the Burns Unit, about the move and what to expect. Starting to like John a bit more. At 2.30 pm, we had the big move down to Burns. Said goodbye to a lot of people. Hope we don't come back – too many bugs floating around up there. Scott took photos of our move and Caro started setting up Sophie's room with her posters, etc. Met the nurses on duty and here we are.

Got to dinner time and we started to wonder how we are going to do it all. Who sleeps where? How do we eat? I came up with the plan that two stay with the girls, i.e. Carolyn and Caroline, while Scott and I go back and cook. We bring back the food, then I go back to the room and eat and babysit Mitchell and Lilly. Tomorrow night will be Scott's turn and I will sleep with Sophie.

Letter to Sophie, Day 50, Friday 6 February 2004
You and I sleep in till 10 am; you keep sleeping till 12 noon. And so you should: only three or four hours of sleep in the last twenty-four mean you are heading for a stress overload.

Dad went with you for your first dressing in the Burns ward; he said your little arms were so thin. There is not as much of the thumb as we thought. I'm so sad for you, my beautiful girl, but I pray that you have a wonderful life – as I know you will.

I leave you resting this afternoon. Ron is in with you this evening, as is Catherine. You have quite a few visitors – Nana and Nanu [Grandmother and Grandfather Delezio], Manuel and Carmen [Ron's brother and sister], Antoni [Catherine Delezio's son] and Louise [Palmer, friend]. I hope it doesn't unsettle you too much. You had pasta for dinner. The nurses expect parents to have an active role in your care, which I will enjoy. You did great physio and proudly announced, 'Mummy, I bent my knees.' Your rectal tube was taken out and you now wear a nappy, which can get very messy with your bandages. You haven't spontaneously laughed for weeks, although you are getting cheeky. Last night at 8.30 pm, when the nurses said they would turn you, you said, 'Sleep like Mummy,' and squeezed your eyes shut.

Carolyn's journal, Day 50, Friday 6 February 2004
We moved Sophie yesterday. Fear, anxiety and sadness were the emotions I felt on leaving ICU. Lonely is what I felt on arriving

out of Intensive Care

at Burns. We had 'lived' in an intensive-care ward for two months – we had experienced the full range of human emotions during this time with doctors and nurses. They had seen us raw and embattled, strong and courageous. They seem distant now, somehow, as we progress with the rehabilitation phase in Sophie's care.

I write these diaries and I know my spelling is appalling; my brain does not yet function to full capacity. I have resigned my position in the company and will not proceed with the purchase – my dream is dead. I will choose a new path for Sophie's sake. I would have loved to do it all but I have to give a hundred and ten per cent to Sophie's care and managing the care and rehabilitation of our family unit through this time. I feel very sad today – a blue sad. I'm tired after sleeping with Sophie, who settled at 4 am. I'm disappointed Sophie doesn't have more of a thumb to create a pincer grip with her right hand. My poor, beautiful daughter. How can you put a price on the life she has lost?

We now face the battle of getting her mobile so her kidneys don't fail as well as her liver. Sophie is not saturating as well as she could and her pulse rate fluctuates a lot with anxiety levels. All I want to do is hold her and tell her that Mummy will make it all better – and I can't. I'm unable to perform the fundamental role of a mother and it leaves me with a deep, gaping wound in my heart.

Ron's journal, Day 50, Friday 6 February 2004
Poor Sophie had a rough night last night. She was up until 2 am, then slept until 3 am, and then was awake until 4 am. She then slept until around 1 pm, when we woke her with a bowel flush. What a disaster. The tube had come out and we were pumping poo all over the place. As if that wasn't bad enough, it went all over her dressings.

Caro's turn to care for Sophie tonight. Had dinner with the

Woods and Beth, who supplied chicken for dinner. Mitchell was very upset about not sleeping with his mum. Had to go back and get Caro to spend a bit of time with him until he slept.

We decided to put a nappy on Sophie. Soph was telling us 'no nappy, no nappy', as she has not had a nappy during the day for a long time.

Letter to Sophie, Day 51, Saturday 7 February 2004
You've had a very restless night. Daddy got about one hour's sleep and you not much more. We have had to put you on a very strict timetable in consultation with Dr Andy and the staff here, because your day/night awareness has been lost due to your time in PICU. There is a specific term for it but I've lost it from my memory bank at present.

This afternoon, when we went to put you prone, your dressings were very green, so I became anxious again. Dr Andy was called and your dressings were promptly removed, with three nurses and him at the helm. Your skin on your back looked good, though the severity of your injuries hit me hard. I became very sad.

Your temp spiked at 40.6 today, which was another fright, so you are now back on antibiotics. You have started eating solids and you crave chicken bones and pasta. You have eighteen hours of feeds and six hours of water. This seems to have helped your demands for water and ice all the time.

Ron's journal, Day 51, Saturday 7 February 2004
What a night. It was my turn to spend the night with Sophie. Got to bed around ten last night with Sophie wide awake. Was kept up all night, due either to Sophie's high temperatures or Sophie demanding water or a chicken bone. During the day, we ended up with our record temperature at 40.6 degrees. Did the

usual things – ice all around her, using the fan and, of course, drugs. Got the temp down and found she had *Pseudomonas* all over her back. Decided to call Andy in for a look.

He got the nurses to remove the Exu-Dry dressing and we called him back in. I really didn't want to see her back again but this time had a look at her tummy as well. I helped them roll Sophie over to check both sides. I found it really hard. How many times do we have to face reality in this place? How many times a day do we cry for Sophie? Seeing the skin is hard enough. What is worse is seeing what Sophie is going through, how much she has suffered and how much she has yet to suffer. I love her so much; my heart is broken into pieces for her. Caro had to come in with us to help emotionally with Sophie while we were doing the dressing. I ended up outside talking to Linda and I broke down again. It never seems to get any easier. I have turned to God so many times for help, for Sophie, Mitchell and me and Caro, and I still can't figure out why He would allow such a thing to happen.

Letter to Sophie, Day 52, Sunday 8 February 2004
You woke every hour last night but slept in between. We started the 'breakfast, nappy change and roll to watch TV on your back' regime. You then have your physio, then go prone, have lunch and sleep time. Afternoon sitting up, stories with friends. Amy, Louise, Beckie and Tricia come to visit from PICU; they are such wonderful nurses.

You want more chicken bones, have some sandwich and pasta for lunch and drink water, but with less intensity.

Your NG [nasogastric] tube to your stomach is removed, as there is less need to aspirate you and you are holding your solids. One less tube – hurray!

Tonight you had fish, rice and chicken on the bone again. Your temp spiked at 40.4 and we had another visit from

PICU – on official business this time at the request of Andy, as your heart rate is up to 202. I get very frightened still at the unexpected changes. My prayers for you to God and Mary MacKillop help me feel like we are not travelling this road alone. I'm very grateful for the wonderful support we have from Andrew, PICU staff and staff of the Burns Unit. The nurses cheered when your NG tube was removed.

Carolyn's journal, Day 52, Sunday 8 February 2004
Anxiety levels high – I fear the central line is playing up. I get fearful and panicked that we may still lose Sophie. It seems like such a long road ahead. Andrew has been in on two or three occasions today already. Sophie is on antibiotics again. I relive the fear of yesterday, when Sophie was going prone and her dressings were green. I had to go out for a walk – doing deep-breathing exercises as hard as I could. 'High panic' is the best way to describe it. I entered her room to see her back looking 'good'. The sheer enormity of her injuries really hits me. My precious, beautiful baby girl. I pray – to calm me and to give me strength to sleep by her side in peace with her. I pray for a restful night for her. My heart is sad as Mitchell goes home today; he left crying and my heart breaks for him.

Ron's journal, Day 52, Sunday 8 February 2004
Woke up with Mitchell and had a bit of a cuddle, got showered and dressed to go and see the girls. Told Caro that we had not eaten yet and she got upset, saying that we should not come over till we are all prepared. Had a bit of an argument and took Mitchell out for breakfast before heading back to Sophie's room. Caro went back to the room with me to sort out Sophie. Decided to turn Sophie on her tummy, or prone, as they say in hospitals. Gave her lunch – some pasta, sandwich and custard, which Sophie ate really well. Just like the old days. Molly was wheeled to the outside of our window so Molly and Sophie

could have a look at each other, with Sophie saying, 'Hello, Molly.' I look forward to taking Sophie outside in the sun; who knows how long it will be until we can do that. Mandy and Maree and Lee came over. It's so much better when people come over during the day; it's too hard at night with taking care of Sophie.

Mitchell and I went to Parramatta Park with Scott and Lilly, then Mandy came to take Mitch to a friend's swimming pool. Margaret the nurse took the clear transpyloric tube out of Sophie's nose today – another milestone for Soph. She's doing really well.

Sophie wanted some 'more bone' (chicken bone), so I went up to KFC and bought one leg. She ate most of it and was very peaceful. Sophie's temp went up during our dinner to 39.6, so back to the ice and fan.

Letter to Sophie, Day 53, Monday 9 February 2004
A great night and sleepy morning, then off to theatre with a central-line issue again; it could be the reason your temp has spiked. Your central line that shouldn't have moved came out by 5 cm. We now have a nurse full-time on line duty when you are turned. You have slept since coming out of theatre at 4.30 pm – it's now 11 pm and I'm finishing off, so I can hopefully get some hours of sleep in before you wake.

I fill your cup because I know you will ask for water sometime soon and hope that you will not ask for a chicken bone.

Andy thinks your back injury is the worst he has seen and is amazed at how well it has healed in only eight weeks. Well done, Sophie.

Carolyn's journal, Day 53, Monday 9 February 2004
Sophie's central line has moved, which sends everyone into a

panic. X-rays and theatre required. I meet [patient] Corey's dad and he puts the fear of God into me about a few nurses as well as the burns bath. I feel panicked and go weak at the knees. A bone in Sophie's right leg may need to be removed due to infection.

Before Sophie goes to theatre, we always sit in the waiting room with her and say a prayer. We go through her bag of icons, which includes a photo of Sophie before her accident and a photo of her now. We sing the 'Beautiful Girl' song [which Carolyn made up for Sophie] and we tell Sophie that we are with her always and will never, ever let her hand go.

When Andy rang after theatre, I thought something must be wrong. We went to the recovery ward for the first time, my heart panicking and my nerves racing. Andy told me prior to theatre that Sophie's back was the worst burn injury he has seen. Peter Hayward said it was the worst head injury he had seen from burns, so all in all it was a great day . . .

Away for ten minutes to pick up a cross from our room. When I got back, Sophie had pooed herself and spiked a temp. I'm going to bed in a tired and nervous state, holding my cross for comfort.

I missed two out of three meetings today, despite remembering them in the morning.

Ron's journal, Day 53, Monday 9 February 2004
Sophie is booked into theatre about 12.30 pm. At 8.30 am, she is sleeping peacefully still. I will wake her soon and start the schedule of getting her ready. We adjust the bed so Sophie is sitting up and then wash her teeth and clean her eyes and cream her face and put her lipstick on [all part of Sophie's pre-theatre ritual to help her feel ready to face another procedure]. Then the wait begins again.

Sophie ended up going in at 1.30 pm to have a dressing change, check the Broviac line and insert a new line for her urine catheter and nasogastric tube. Taking Sophie into theatre is always hard. I have the same routine every time. I get Sophie to tell me that she is a big, strong girl, louder and louder, as loud as she can just before she gets her injection. I then give her a kiss and tell her that I love her just before she goes to sleep. Then I walk back to the waiting room to be with Carolyn.

Had some lunch at the restaurant and ended up speaking to Rod Smith about the court case.

Everyone keeps on saying how inspirational we are. I don't think this way – we do what we have to do because we have no choice. We do, however, do our best for Sophie and Mitchell. Sophie is the brave one. She is the one feeling all the pain. She is the one who doesn't even know she has lost her legs, fingers and ear. She is the one who has smiled without prompting maybe a dozen times in the last eight weeks. I still can't understand how she manages to smile at all under these circumstances.

Caro and I were in Sophie's room when Andy rang from theatre saying that the Broviac line was a bit messy with infection, the same as the end of her right leg. Caro, as expected, was in a panic about this. Anyway, Sophie was being sent back down to the recovery ward and we were taken up there to meet her. Sophie was still asleep when Andy came in to talk. He said that if her high temperatures continued, he would remove the Broviac line and insert another arterial line, as she had before. Next, he told us that he covered the end of her right leg with Acticoat [antimicrobial barrier dressing] and that if it did not clear the infection he would remove the other bone – not her tibia but a smaller bone. He said that she did not need it to accept a prosthesis. It's still another kick in the guts. Fancy telling someone you don't need a bone in your leg. Anyway, he was concerned but not overly concerned.

Got back to the room and spoke to Sandra about things and the phone just kept on ringing. I switched it off. Couldn't handle it any more. Catherine came for an hour or so and held

Sophie's hand and set up her bed with her toys. The nurses came in, as I told them we needed to turn her onto her tummy. We thought it was best while she was still out of it. I discussed with the nurses that in future we need to have a nurse just to watch her lines, as we can't afford for them to be pulled again. This worked fine.

Letter to Sophie, Day 54, Tuesday 10 February 2004
A sleepy morning after a very big sleep for the second night. It's wonderful – I hope the routine continues to work. You were never able to settle in PICU with all the activity – I know you always just wanted to be a part of the party. Andy often referred to it as the party place. Issues remain on what to do with temps, central line and the next graft. Andy is in consultation with Peter. Amy from PICU visits, as do Lee, Mum and Louise, all armed with stories and activities. Your physio starts in earnest, with you seated at forty-five degrees, with rolls under your bottom so you don't slide down your bed. You have tomato soup and stewed apple today – you have never eaten tomatoes, so I was surprised when you finished the plate of soup.

We will try a routine for you again tomorrow – you seem to like the pattern. Your feeds will go in overnight, so we can start to finger feed you during the day. Gustave the mouse puppet drops in when you do good physio; you look at him rather strangely but it keeps your mind off your discomfort. You received a beautiful quilt from some ladies at Scone; it has rainbows and bubbles around the edge – very appropriate for all the sending of rainbows and blowing of bubbles we do.

Carolyn's journal, Day 54, Tuesday 10 February 2004
I met with Sandra to explain my confusion at times and get reassurance about the upside for serious-burns survivors and

their passage. She reminded me to take one day at a time and not dwell on the negatives. I want to meet some inspirational people to help me get some positive outlooks on this journey, where the light at times seems so distant. Sophie's care seems all-consuming to me.

Ron's journal, Day 54, Tuesday 10 February 2004
Woke up around 6 am, as Caro was sleeping with Sophie and wanted to go to t'ai chi class. Stayed with Sophie till 8 am, then headed home to take Mitchell to school. Mitch was looking for worms with Grandpa Allan. He was very excited about seeing me, as well as spotting some lizards on the way. Walked to school with Mitch; it was great to hold his hand again. I miss Mitchell very much. He has grown so much that I feel I have missed out on a lot. Fiona [Jiggins, director of Mitchell's preschool] said that a new boy started yesterday and that Mitchell took care of him all day. Very proud of him.

Went to Dr Chris for a check-up, as my throat was sore from the night before with Sophie. The air conditioning is very cold and very strong. Dr Chris took my blood pressure and said it was extremely high. Had a look at my throat and prescribed some penicillin. Did some banking and got back to the hospital at 4.30 pm.

Letter to Sophie, Day 55, Wednesday 11 February 2004
I heard that John Laws and Alan Jones talked about you on radio today. You had a visit from Captain Starlight [one of a team of Starlight captains who entertain children in hospital], who sang 'Twinkle Twinkle', 'Old MacDonald' and 'The Lion Sleeps Tonight' to you. You sang along to 'Old MacDonald', then, when he blew you a kiss, you blew one back to him. He sent a message out to the Starlight Foundation saying he got a kiss from you!

You needed blood and oxygen today, and some lung specialists to keep you well for your next op on Friday. You have a partial collapse of the lung again. We got you sitting up in bed today at about forty-five degrees, but any more and your respiratory rate suffered. You are eating more but a little too much tonight: you vomited, so we will cut back on how much you eat – less than three tablespoons. Lyn South, your ward granny, sat with you while you slept, which gave me some time for washing and cleaning, getting our room ready for Mitchell's arrival tonight. Carolyn and Charlotte Reid are bringing him in. It will be nice to be together again. I have this beautiful picture in my mind of 15 December: you, Mitchell and me walking down the steps of our home. You are so pretty in your red checks and shorts and hat, all Christmassy for your party. My beautiful girl.

Carolyn's journal, Day 55, Wednesday 11 February 2004
I saw Sophie's arms on video today – broken body, broken limbs, loss of innocence. Captain Starlight sent an email to the whole Starlight Foundation saying he got a kiss from Sophie. I cried.

No sitting up in Sophie's special seat – no physio. Chest X-rays and chest specialists instead. Sophie has a collapsed lung, chest infection, blood transfusion, haemoglobins down, and swelling in her left arm needing bandages; her cut-off arm must be raised in a splint for three additional hours and elevated overnight.

Ron's journal, Day 55, Wednesday 11 February 2004
Had a meeting with Sandra this afternoon. We talked about what's going on and how I was feeling. I told her about going to the doctor yesterday and she advised me that if things were getting too hard I could go on medication (antidepressants). I told Sandra that I was coping most of the time but that I felt

overwhelmed by the whole experience. We seem to be getting somewhere, but it seems an endless journey and I am not sure that I can cope. I feel as though I am breaking apart and am all alone. Sandra said it was a good idea to consider antidepressants if and when I thought the time was right. I said that I thought the time was getting closer. I agreed to talk to the psychiatrist next week. It scares me thinking that I may be on antidepressants. I have heard about so many side effects.

Letter to Sophie, Day 56, Thursday 12 February 2004
Congratulations, you are a star! You sat in a chair this morning and blew lots of bubbles in a bottle – like volcanoes. It was a big effort but you did really well; it was after a big cuddle on Dad's lap. I think it will be my turn tomorrow. You had a blood transfusion again today and you had your legs bathed. You are also wrapped in your Exu-Dry coat and you look so neat and tidy. Your arm is better after having had your bandages loosened because your fingers were swelling. They looked a bit blue but now they have warmth in them again and a pink hue. You wanted a Wiggles Band-Aid on your thumb where the nail and tip are black. Your new nail is growing through, just the same as Dad's on his thumb. You are looking peaceful after an unsettled period following your dressing change. Your stats are 98 oxygen saturation and 138 ECG – the lowest I've ever seen it.

Carolyn's journal, Day 56, Thursday 12 February 2004
I feel like I have achieved something – I got one phone call out during the day! Met with Mary re work, which was a godsend. She is running the business till June – I have withdrawn my interest. Mitchell met with Sandra, and Sophie sat in a chair today – it's taken since Monday to get her in it, because of all the unscheduled complications. Another day just disappeared

between attending to Sophie and time with Mitchell and his demands, which are many. I dropped him off at kindy crying today because he didn't want to stay – but I needed it. He did too, though he had only been with us overnight. I have slept with Sophie six nights and I am tired – the broken-sleep issue reminds me of breastfeeding and holding an infant.

Ron's journal, Day 56, Thursday 12 February 2004
Sophie had a good night's sleep, with groups of three to four hours between waking up. Did all the usual things and then sat Sophie up for breakfast. Sophie ate a poached egg and some Rice Bubbles. Then I had Soph on my lap for a little while. Had a great cuddle with Soph and we sang 'Rock-a-Bye Baby' a number of times. After this, we sat her in a special seat, which we put on the bed. She looked great sitting up there. Sang some more songs before putting her prone to go to sleep before lunch.

Later, had Sophie blow the party whistles. She was great. Just wanted to keep on going until she was exhausted! Caro needed to post some letters in Westmead Hospital and I wanted the three of us to go. Caro just took her time so I left them to it. I had the shits.

The washing of Sophie's left and possibly right leg was booked for 2 pm in the ward. Ended up happening around 3 pm. Caro came in with me but ended up going back out before they removed the bandages. Sandra also came in for support. It's probably the third time that I have seen an amputated leg and the first time that I have looked at the end of an amputated leg, let alone that of my own daughter. Her left leg was already covered with grafted skin and everyone was saying how good it looked. I could not see much difference. I keep on wondering how much Sophie can handle. It looks so horrific, with burns all over her tiny legs. I said to David (anaesthetist), 'It's now over eight weeks and this is what it still looks like?' It just goes to show how bad it must have been eight weeks ago. I cried a lot and held myself together a lot. It's so hard seeing your little baby like this. She must be so strong and has yet to be so strong for such a long time. Back in the room now, writing this and looking at Sophie. She is so beautiful, just lying there.

chapter five
under pressure

Two months on, the stress is starting to show. For Ron and Carolyn, the unrelieved fear, ongoing exposure to their daughter's pain, and sheer sleep deprivation translate into short tempers and intolerance – between themselves and with the nursing staff.

Mitchell, too, is acting out his frustration. Only four and a half years old, he has a massive load to bear: deprived of his parents' attention and care, spending large slabs of time in the alien environment of the hospital, and exposed to a crisis that he can barely comprehend.

None of us knows what the future holds, but for Sophie's family at this point in their lives the days and years ahead must seem both unfathomable and bleak.

Letter to Sophie, Day 57, Friday 13 February 2004
You had your right leg grafted today. Your central line stayed put; there are not many options in terms of sites, so while no

infection is present the surgeons say it is best to leave well enough alone. You did not need to go to PICU and we are so glad you came through the op with flying colours.

Chris and Vere [Sharma, friends] came over from New Zealand to see you today. So did Russell, Dad's friend from schooldays, whose son was burnt twenty years ago. The emotion for him is still there; he said his visit was like déjà vu. He told us some stories about difficult situations that we know in time we will face, but we know your sunny personality and open outlook will guide you through.

I held you in my arms today before you sat on your seat and it was wonderful. I felt so privileged to have you in my arms, and I was so full of love for you.

You blew your new recorder with big, deep breaths. Grandma Joy found it for you – it has all the colours of the rainbow and we played 'Baa Baa Black Sheep' together. Lyn, your ward granny, sat with you while Ron and I had a bite of lunch together, which is often the only time we get to talk to each other about life outside hospital.

Carolyn's journal, Day 57, Friday 13 February 2004
Stress city – Burns are down one nurse because they thought ICU would have Sophie after her graft. Ron can't understand why I want Sophie's bed elevated; it's for drainage of her lung and he's getting all hot tempered after she comes out of recovery. I arrived back at our room at 9 pm, leaving Ron to sort out feeds and catch up on drugs for Sophie. Mitchell is jumping on the bed. Thank goodness Chris and Vere were here to help get things sorted with Mitchell and Lilly – baths, dinner, etc.

I eat with Caroline and Scott – Ron in with Sophie. Chris and Vere make a fast exit. Other than the high-stress environment, Sophie's graft on her leg went well.

Our environment seems surreal. The bad-dream embers re-emerge and life seems stilted.

Ron's journal, Day 57, Friday 13 February 2004

Haven't been able to sleep the last couple of nights – only getting around two or three hours a night. Have been taking sleeping tablets but they have been useless. I think it's been because I have been seeing Sophie's arms and legs recently for dressing and I have been very disturbed over it. Caro and I have not been getting on. She gets irritated with me and I with her. We both speak badly to each other. I feel the pressure getting to us both.

At around 4 am, I woke from a broken sleep to find Mitchell on top of me, asleep. I wish I could have stayed that way for the rest of the morning but I knew I would definitely not be able to sleep that way. God bless him. And God bless Caro. I love them both very, very much. Maybe I do need the antidepressant drugs. I need to talk to Caro about it but my pride keeps getting in the way. I do know what I must do.

Decided to shave and take Mitchell for breakfast before seeing Caro. I don't understand why she doesn't want us to all have breakfast together. I could bring it from the cafe to the room. Stuff her. Went to see Sophie, and Caro left the room. Sophie was fasting from 6 am as she was due in theatre around twelve to have her right leg grafted and possibly her central line changed. She was asleep most of the day anyway – I think from not eating for so long. She had breakfast yesterday morning, then was fasted for lunch due to leg dressing, did not wake for dinner and fasted for theatre from 6 am.

Russell, an old friend, came over. Had some coffee and a talk. Russell's son, Aaron, was badly burnt around twenty years ago when Aaron's brother filled the bath with boiling water, causing sixty-five-per-cent burns. He is now twenty-one and living a normal life. I must thank Russell for coming out. Rod Smith brought the barrister over. Unfortunately, we didn't have much time to spend with them as they arrived around three and Sophie ended up going to theatre around 4.30 pm.

Sophie's graft went very well. Her right leg is now fully covered and they decided to keep the Broviac line that she had. The old 'kick in the guts' came again when we were talking to Peter about the quarantine. The good news was that there was only fifteen per cent of her body left to cover – the head and other bits and pieces. The kick was that they removed the fibula, the bone in her leg where the infection was found the other day. Another piece of Sophie removed. She's such a brave girl. Why do we complain about trivial things?

Letter to Sophie, Day 58, Saturday 14 February 2004
Your head was dressed today. Daddy and I were in the room with you and we saw your wounds; you have lost your right ear but I was surprised at how neat it looked – I'm not sure what I was expecting. You handled the dressing change very well.

You were a little unsettled tonight: you have had extra morphine just to change your nappy. Daddy wasn't happy. Mitchell came up to your bed today and said, 'I love you, Sophie.' I think he will be a very supportive brother to you in your rehabilitation. He blew you kisses and you blew some back. I think we need to arrange your timetable more efficiently – I will be putting thought into that over the next day or so before our weekly meeting with Carrie [Hopwood, nursing-unit manager of the Burns Unit]. Angela Holden, one of your nurses in PICU, came to visit; I wish we had them down here with you all the time.

Carolyn's journal, Day 58, Saturday 14 February 2004
I pine for the good old days of ease – little tension and a happy family life. Today, I have a stressed four-year-old, a stressed husband, I'm stressed and Sophie distressed after the dressing change on her head. Actually, I think Ron is shattered; he said

his legs went weak in the dressing-change room. I'm tired, so tired, and I just want to go home – perhaps I can dream of how things were.

Ron's journal, Day 58, Saturday 14 February 2004
Not a bad night's sleep. Sophie woke up every one to two hours and me accordingly. I had more sleep than I have had in the last two or three days. I must admit it still feels good to hear Sophie calling for Daddy. I love the sound of her voice. I could not live without hearing her and being near her. It makes me think about Sue (who lost her two-month-old, Lucas, two weeks ago) and Chris (who lost her eleven-year-old around four weeks ago). I can't imagine how they felt, losing their children.

During the night, Sophie did a poo. When I sat up, she told me to 'lie down, Daddy' a number of times. Other days, she would say, 'Not me, not me.' She hates getting her nappy changed because of the pain involved. Woke up trying to remember if [nurse X] had been washing her hands on entering and leaving the room. I must keep a closer eye on this as I don't want Sophie getting any more infections.

The dressing session was a disaster. They removed the head dressing and Caro and I saw her entire head, including her missing right ear. I could hardly control myself. Had a meeting with Andy afterwards, who said that we need to work towards dressing in the ward without an anaesthetist. I thought this would take some time. Spent most of the afternoon with Sophie. She did a poo and we had to clean it up. The poor thing was so distressed we had to give her three boluses to calm her down. I think the rectal tube is much better and less distressing for Sophie. Had dinner with the Woods; Caro's turn with Sophie tonight, as my legs are ready to give way.

Letter to Sophie, Day 59, Sunday 15 February 2004
Transpyloric tube blocked – this goes to your lower intestine; it feeds you and is where your drugs are put in. We had three people trying to flush it, including Andy.

You had a dressing change in theatre on two arms, as well as your nappy change. Your right arm is not fully grafted, as we lost some of the skin. Your left arm is healing very well.

You were very tired post-op and needed an oxygen mask again today. Lee brought you the most beautiful pop-up book and Maree brought you in her rainbow sheet and pillowcase. I've put one of your pillows in it and we'll see how you like it. Auntie Michelle and Paul [friend] came to visit today and brought you a Wiggles tape recorder. You've already sung into it, despite it having no batteries. You are my true champion – I love you!

Carolyn's journal, Day 59, Sunday 15 February 2004
I can't believe I still can't get more than one phone call out of this place. I miss Mitchell; he went home with Beth, had a haircut and played at [his friend] Brayden's house. I saw Sophie's arm today at a dressing change. Andy is keen to press on with her schedule of daily changes – it means daily fasting. We will see how her feeds go.

Sophie's hand was so cold from lack of circulation that her probe wouldn't work. Because we had no reading of blood pressure, oxygen saturation, heart rate, they had to massage her hand to warm it before it would read. It took an hour – the hour we were hoping to feed Sophie dinner. And so another day passes.

Ron's journal, Day 59, Sunday 15 February 2004
8 am. As usual, I woke just thinking *here we go again*. I need to get shaved, get Mitchell ready and go over to Sophie's room asap before Caro gets the shits. I slept okay for the first time

in a long time. I think it may be because I am starting to get to grips with going on antidepressants – I'm just getting too cranky nowadays. I'm finding Mitchell is getting more disturbed lately, probably a little more naughty. I can't blame him, with what he's going through. Every time I organise to do something with him, something comes up and it just doesn't happen. That's the thing about priorities: someone ends up getting hurt – in this case, Mitchell.

It was agreed that Sophie was to have her arms dressed around 1–2 pm. I'm sick of the nursing staff saying that it's okay to have just gas [i.e. that there's no need to have an anaesthetist present], and they do it all the time; our nurse checked and found that Sophie had not been certified to be gassed by just Burns nurses. So Doc Andy agreed to be there during the procedure if an anaesthetist was present in the ward at the time.

Strange how I am getting used to seeing Sophie's burns and not feeling so distressed. Took some more photos and the dressing was over. Came back to the room, then went over to see Rod Smith about legal matters. Discussed the charity set-up and all is cool. Went back to Sophie's room and found she was very sluggish. All the nurses agreed that Sophie was 'plumb tuckered out'. Sat Sophie up and she seemed a lot better. I had to take food out of her mouth for fear that she would end up choking on it. They stopped the morphine because she was too out of it. She picked up a bit and we were very relieved.

Went back for dinner around 9 pm and made the offer to Scott and family that if they have to leave their rental property, they can stay in our home until they buy a place. I'm not too sure at this stage when they would leave the hospital, but the offer was there and they were happy to accept. Back to Sophie's room, where I am in charge tonight. Let's hope it's a good night. Good night all.

Letter to Sophie, Day 60, Monday 16 February 2004
I held you today. You were doing yoga exercises, going up on your shoulders with your legs in the air to have your nappy changed. In theatre today, I told you stories about the ginger cat. We have also started cutting dressings for Tricia, your doll. She wears a splint and, whatever you are having done, Tricia gets it too! Tonight, after your zinc supplement, you threw up. Big-time dressing had to be cut away. You sang beautifully into your tape recorder today, in between your oxygen. You asked Catherine to come and visit and she did; you two have a very special bond. I will never forget her for sleeping by your side for the first couple of weeks. You love your sleep routine and we are so thankful that you love it too – you wake up every one to three hours but rest again quickly.

Carolyn's journal, Day 60, Monday 16 February 2004
We arrive to find Sophie with a temperature of 40.6 degrees; it had not been checked for three hours. This was just after 9 am. When we asked why it was not taken every hour, one nurse said, 'We couldn't do or give her anything more anyway.' I said, 'Yes you can – ice, the fan on and a phone call to us and the doctor.' I disassociate myself from what was then to what is now and I focus on the task at hand: to get my baby back and healthy and to cradle her in my arms. It is so sad.

Ron's journal, Day 60, Monday 16 February 2004
Not a bad night with Sophie. Had two-hour stretches at times. At 8 am, I went back to the room and had a shower, etc. before going back to Sophie. She had a temp of 40.6 degrees. The nurse was asked when the last temp was taken; she looked it up and said three hours ago. I said Sophie was supposed to have her temp taken every hour. The nurse said in a smart way, 'Well, okay. I couldn't do anything anyway,' and walked out. I followed her to the front desk and had a go at her, telling her

that I expected Sophie to be checked every hour and that Sophie was my main concern and I didn't want to deal with a person with an attitude like hers.

Sophie had low stats all day and was being fasted for an 11 am leg dressing. The dressing went well and I carried Sophie back to the room, where we put her prone and she went to sleep. We then had a (weekly) meeting in the long-stay room. Cath from across the courtyard advised us all that she was leaving on Sunday. I went and had a look at her room; it is better than ours and it has its own courtyard area at the back. We agreed that we would have it on Sunday if they moved out.

Spoke to Richard [Smith, Day of Difference director] about Allan's car: arranging a swap with Toyota in New Zealand for a new car in Australia. Another job off my plate. Went back to Sophie, and Catherine was there. We had some fun singing songs with Sophie on video. Her spirits were starting to rise as the temperatures were going down. Sophie had a bit of green (infection) on her outfit. Andy said he would have a look at it tomorrow and decide what to do. Not sure what to do, as I had arranged to take Mitchell to school in the morning.

Letter to Sophie, Day 61, Tuesday 17 February 2004
Your NG tube blocked today and you needed a new one. You are so brave, as you swallow when it passes through your throat to your stomach. You are handling your feeds well.

This evening, we took you outside for the first time, strapped to a wheelchair in a reclining seat. You looked frail sitting under Nana's blanket with baby Tricia sitting on your knee.

We had a big meeting today with all the staff about your condition and what affects you most. We've formulated a plan and hope you will adapt – we will adapt around you in terms of dressing changes and rectal tubes (we must remember lemonade iceblocks when the nappy is changed!). Your case is so complicated that each day if we get half the scheduled physio done, we feel as though we have achieved something.

Carolyn's journal, Day 61, Tuesday 17 February 2004
I'm sad. Ron's sad. Ron's in tears. This afternoon, we tried to get Sophie outside and succeeded, but within forty-five minutes her temp had gone from 37.7 to 40.6 degrees. She was listless and half-asleep in the chair but didn't want to go in. My beautiful girl looked like a total invalid, covered in a crocheted blanket with her head on one side as she had no strength to hold her head up. What should have been a joyous moment was sad and painful because she didn't have the spirit or strength to enjoy it.

Ron's journal, Day 61, Tuesday 17 February 2004
The morning started off at around 5 am. Woke up thinking about things and tossing and turning. Eventually, got up at 7 am to check on Sophie before I went home. Had a quick meeting with Dr Andy and Caro in Sophie's room. Discussed leaving her dressing until tomorrow. Drove home with Mitchell's new slot-car set. Mitch opened his car set, all excited. He cuddled me hard and fully. I could feel his loneliness and sadness. I also knew that five minutes into being at day care with his friends he would be happy again. I cried as I walked out the school gate.

Walked back home and took Allan to the hairdressers for a cut. After I had my haircut too, I went and saw Erica [real-estate agent] and she told me about a house on Seaforth Crescent, which is for sale. The house hasn't been lived in for ten years. Took Allan for a look. At 1350 m^2, it is almost twice the size of our existing block. Fair views, though not great, but a big block – very overgrown. Spoke to Rod Smith on the phone about barristers, etc. and he told me that Mikala [his daughter] was very excited about coming out to read to Sophie.

Left home and went back to our 'other home' at the hospital for the 3.15 meeting with all the staff teams: pain, infections, physio, nurses, and Dr Andy. Agree that Friday's dressing change will be with an anaesthetist and Monday's dressing change for the arms and legs will be with just gas. Worth a try. That night, when I was with Sophie, I realised how sad I was.

Letter to Sophie, Day 62, Wednesday 18 February 2004
Today, you went to theatre and had a dressing change: everything is looking good with your grafts. You were cold when you came out so needed to stay in recovery for longer than last time. You have been given a cortisone cream for your face; we were concerned a rash was spreading from your grafts to your nose. You have a yeast infection in the blood. Your left arm and index finger are in plaster so your finger can straighten. You had lots of physio in theatre and one of your Burns nurses was up there to see you so they can be better prepared in the burns baths [special area for burns dressing changes] on the wards.

Our plan is to try to have dressing changes every two to four days so you are not under gas or sedation every day. We need to concentrate on your bubble-blowing, music and lung-expansion exercises so that you can breathe again without the mask.

We hope to have you in the chair again tomorrow, so we want you happy and well to do that. Tonight, I hope you have a settled sleep, seeing as you only had three hours of solid sleep yesterday. It was Dad's turn to sleep with you; he got one hour and was not impressed.

Carolyn's journal, Day 62, Wednesday 18 February 2004
Big arguments with Ron tonight – I'm not sure what about but he is really stressed. Accused me of not caring when I took an

hour off to play mah-jong. I had been in Sophie's room twenty-two of the previous twenty-four hours. Irrational of Ron, I think. It's exhausting and tempers fray easily.

I picked Mitchell up today and went home. I find my mind contemplates the accident all the time when I drive. I drove past the M3 exit, so had to go to Chatswood and take the M2.

Ron's journal, Day 62, Wednesday 18 February 2004
What a night. Didn't hit the pillow until around 2 am and from then it was up every half-hour as Sophie was upset and distressed. She would wake up, grimacing; not sure whether it was nightmares or pain. Either way, she was obviously distressed. Around 6 am, Sophie decided to go to sleep. I let her sleep until around 9 am, as we had to get ready for a dressing change in theatre. During this time, we bought some coffee and met up with Russell and Janice and Allan and Joy, then we went and waited in the waiting room for Sophie to finish up. We were called in to see Sophie in an anaesthetic state (very drowsy, and moving all the time). Caro left after that and went to pick up Mitchell, and I stayed with Sophie the rest of the day. Had a half-hour massage at 3.30 pm – a pretty light one but still relaxing. When Caro arrived, I took Mitchell to the cafe and fed him before going back to our room and having dinner with Scott and Caroline. I discussed Scott's QC representing us and there are no hassles at all. Had a fight with Caro about I don't know what and she kept on telling me to go on antidepressants as a way of getting back at me. Caro left to go and take care of Sophie, and that was it for the night.

Letter to Sophie, Day 63, Thursday 19 February 2004
My darling girl, I left you for five hours so I could advise my staff that I was resigning. It was difficult being away from you

and I felt anxious to get back. I know you were in good hands. Mum and Dad were on deck, as well as Lee and Mark, to help care for you and Mitchell. Trudy visited also, with baby in tum! You put your hand on Trudy's tum and felt the baby move. Trudy asked us to be its godparents – how wonderful!

You had a better day, the first 'good day' since you have been on the ward. A big sleep till noon and another good sleep this afternoon. You had a big appetite, too, and I hear you were blowing bubbles and your sparkling personality was showing through.

You ate a bowl and a half of soup tonight, and doctors who haven't seen you for a week or so are saying you have put on weight in your face. I just love to know your spirit is soaring, because that gives me hope beyond all else. You are our star and you are the luckiest girl to have such a caring, compassionate brother in Mitchell, who at times struggles with not being with us and with the attention that you receive from everyone.

Carolyn's journal, Day 63, Thursday 19 February 2004
I feel like a displaced person today – not because I told the staff I resigned but because I was driving along, looking at life outside a children's hospital and wondering what it is all about. Being incredibly sad about what has happened to our little girl and questioning what the future holds. We will be forever grateful for having the companionship and friendship of the Wood family through this shocking period in our lives.

Ron's journal, Day 63, Thursday 19 February 2004
Woke up with Mitchell – always a nice way to wake up. Thought to myself it would be nice for Mitch to roll over and give me a cuddle. I kept on reaching across and patting his shoulder but he wouldn't take the hint. God bless him! We ended up going to breakfast with me thinking, *wouldn't it be nice if I could shave and shower and get dressed, then take Mitchell to the cafe and*

buy breakfast to take over to Sophie's room so we could all have breakfast together. But unfortunately Caro gets upset when I get there without being ready to take over.

Letter to Sophie, Day 64, Friday 20 February 2004
Peter and Andy came round and saw you sitting in your chair today. Peter wants you tubeless in three weeks so you can have a break from your central line. He has a plan for you to be fully grafted in four weeks. He thinks you may be ready for prosthetic limbs in three months. I dream of the day I can take you home. I had the most beautiful hold of you today and didn't want to let you go but you had to go prone. I just wanted the moment to last forever – you are my beautiful girl.

You blew bubbles with Catherine and Daddy this evening. I think we need to get in at least three sets of half-hour blowing exercises per day so that you can go off oxygen.

Problems with your probe tonight when your hands get cold again – you lose circulation in your fingers and your monitor doesn't read. You only have two fingers available for your probe, so there aren't many options.

Carolyn's journal, Day 64, Friday 20 February 2004
Another day disappears. Mitchell is rebelling by wanting to be carried all the time, kicking, punching and biting me. Sophie is so sleepy it's hard to accomplish anything like the physio we need to do on her chest to enable her to breathe on her own again. It's as if she is doing catch-up from the last two months in ICU. We manage to get the splints on and to have her prone. Just enough time for a small amount of food and stories. And, again, I only manage one phone call. I need a couple of hours to tidy up work stuff on Monday and maybe move house.

chapter six
'I do not want to lose her'

In late February, the Delezios begin planning their house move, looking at places that can be adapted for Sophie's particular needs. Increasingly, what they want to find is a house that will be Sophie's 'house for life': a home that will accommodate her intense and very specific physical requirements. Eventually, they decide to build a house in Balgowlah Heights, but from making that decision their home takes eighteen months to plan and two years to build.

Very soon after Sophie's accident, Ron and Carolyn resolved not to shy away from the publicity that surrounded their private tragedy. In their eyes, if Sophie's story brought hope or inspiration to others, something good would have emerged from their suffering. Accordingly, they decide to allow a 60 Minutes crew to film Sophie with her doctors, friends, therapists and family.

All of their dreams and plans, though, are put on hold once again on Day 65, when Sophie becomes gravely ill.

Letter to Sophie, Day 65, Saturday 21 February 2004
You are not well – pale and listless, your breathing is laboured. PICU are called and a decision is made after consistent high temps the night before to move you to ICU. Dad and I are in tears, because you have fought so hard to get to the Burns Unit, but your breathing is going backward, not forward. It's very scary and sad but we know you are going to be in the best hands and in a way it is a relief to know that two doctors will be on hand in the neighbouring room.

You are fitted with a fluid bolus and albumin to rehydrate you and pumped with antibiotics. Your central line is removed and a new femoral line [inserted in the groin area] is introduced. You were septic. We are anxious for you. Andy checked your back and there was an area that was infected due to poo. A decision was made to take you to theatre to do your dressings on Monday. You are placed prone from about 6 pm, to remain that way till morning. Tonight, we can sleep with Mitchell, who this morning asked when we could all sleep together in the room. He misses you and gets a bit cranky about being here but mostly is good, with diversions from friends.

Ron's journal, Day 65, Saturday 21 February 2004
John [Stewart] rang to say he was in the foyer and that Caro was still asleep. Rang Caro to get her up and I shaved, showered and dressed before going down to Sophie's room. Sophie is getting weaker and weaker. John left and we got down to business. Sophie's haemoglobin is down to 8.3; the last time her haemoglobin was down, she got weak as well. That time, within one hour of her transfusion she was fine. The ICU team came down and did more blood tests, and her haemoglobin was 8.5, which was okay. They did all the other tests too. By then, Sophie could hardly speak; her heart rate was over two hundred and they could not get it down. A few more doctors came down and we all agreed that Sophie should go back up to ICU.

We had dreaded the day that Sophie might have to go back there. We held each other tight, scared for her. We packed up Sophie's bed, took all the bears and dolls and left Trish and baby. We began our journey out of Burns to ICU, being careful to put the blanket on Sophie, as we were aware of stares from some people. Up in the lifts to the third floor. God, I didn't want to come here. I thought things would have to be bad for us to come back up here.

Got Sophie into bed and they gave her some albumin, and she perked up straight away. Her colour came back, her breathing was good, she was talking again. Wow – what a relief. The registrars, Stephen and Amish, decided it was time to fit a new central line. They used ketamine for the procedure. Amish tried to get access on her right side first – no luck. We then tried the left side a couple of times. I was starting to worry it was going to turn out to involve something a bit more serious, like having to go back to theatre. They went back to her right side again – success. They had a good fix in her vein. Sophie was just so great during the procedure. Half an hour later, Sophie spread both her arms out and said to me, 'I'm flying, I'm flying – shhhhhhhh.' I was lucky enough to have my camera with me, so I filmed the flying event on video. This will be great on her twenty-first birthday.

Tonight is a special night: Caro and Mitch and I can spend the night together.

Letter to Sophie, Day 66, Sunday 22 February 2004
You have a staph infection in the blood. You have to be intubated again, which will give your lungs time to recuperate. Because of all the fluid pumped into you yesterday, your lungs are saturated. You will not go prone today because you still have fluid behind your eyes. Sister Bridget came to see you today, as

did Dave and Mary and Mandy, who spent time with Mitchell. We move into another long-stay unit with a balcony – we can now look at some greenery. You are very sleepy; your morphine has been increased, your feeds stopped and recommenced later in the evening. You will be fasted again tomorrow for theatre, so we will try to get as much food into you overnight and in the morning as we can. You need regular physio and you are on significant antibiotics but your temperature hasn't really spiked as high as the last few days. I want you to rest easy, my baby, so your body can have a break from trying so hard to fight all the infections. You are our precious baby girl.

Ron's journal, Day 66, Sunday 22 February 2004
Woke up late. First night together for three weeks. I went up to see Sophie and found she was still asleep. Caro and Mitch were moving house downstairs. Sophie was still weak and Amish said that we should let her sleep and rest. Andy came in around 10 am and we fitted the rectal tube. I asked Andy to check her dressing. Andy pulled up her dressing and found poo on the back of it, with pus all over a three-by-two area. Cleaned it up and redressed her.

Left her to sleep till around 4 pm, when I returned to find Caro with Sophie, saying that she may need to be intubated and that because of low oxygen saturation a different mask had to be fitted. They advised that Sophie had a staph infection in her blood and that more results were needed but that they had given her a broad range of antibiotics to cover everything they could think of. They did another X-ray, which showed her lower left lung was a little collapsed and there was moisture in another large part of her lung. They had given Soph some diuretics, as the fluid was staying inside and needed to get out. We'll see what happens. Tonight, Sophie is very sedated and will sleep well.

Letter to Sophie, Day 67, Monday 23 February 2004

It's an early night for us: we are both sitting writing our diaries at 10 pm. It's quite different with you being in PICU with your own nurse. They will make the decisions for you for the next two weeks on the ward. We have been calling the shots a lot and getting things done that needed to be pushed. Your day started with a new tube being needed: they had to extubate, then intubate again to get the new tube down. You have been fasted for three days because of all the procedures, so again we play catch-up.

You are very heavily sedated; you require four times the usual dose for the intubation today. Your antifungal meds are increased with possible toxic outcomes, so you will be carefully monitored, especially by me. Your dressing change was done in the ward because Andy wanted you to stay put, eliminating the need to change your ventilator. He was pleased with what he saw. I pray tonight that your little body gets the rest it so desperately needs so that I can again see your spirit shine through. You have so many doctors and nurses popping in to visit and wanting to work with you again. Everyone wants you to get through this so they can see you shine at the other end – the light at the end of the tunnel. I want to hold you again like I did yesterday. My big, brave girl. I love you and pray God will keep you safe.

Ron's journal, Day 67, Monday 23 February 2004

The nurses said Sophie had an easy night and that her oxygen levels are getting less dependent on the ventilator. They planned to replace this tube at 11.30 am and to do a complete dressing with a Burns nurse. I felt lost, not knowing what to do with myself. Sophie was sleeping with sedation and I couldn't do anything for her, so I decided to go to Westfield and do some shopping for things I needed.

Came back and the intubation was done, and she was still resting nicely. Did a few things on the computer and made a few phone calls and had a cup of coffee. Had a phone call from Caro saying that she went up to Sophie's room and they were doing the dressing change without a Burns nurse. I met her and went to the Burns ward; nurse Dianne said she was still waiting for ICU to let her know when Sophie was ready. Caro was very upset. I went up to Sophie's room and Andy arrived and helped with the head and the back. Took some photos and everything seemed fine. Spoke to Amish, who said they were happy with Sophie's progress and that they had decided to get a lot more aggressive with the medication for Sophie's finger infection.

Met up with Lee and Catherine, and we all had coffee, followed by a visit to Sophie. Spoke to Cliff Neville, one of the *60 Minutes* producers – we have had dinner at his house a couple of times. [Cliff is a friend of Carolyn's parents, Joy and Allan.] He suggested that we have an informal meeting this week and he would get a $ figure from Channel 9 as a donation to Sophie and Molly's trust fund. I spoke to Trudy and said that any approach to *60 Minutes* should now go through Cliff and he would involve the other directors that did the Bali story with him. He suggested that he could bring Peter Overton and I said if this were the case we would need to meet at another venue, as too many people would recognise Peter and I didn't want to attract attention. He agreed. I told Trudy to organise things for next Thursday, even though Sophie was to be in theatre for her head graft.

I went up to see Sophie later and Caro told me that they had to replace the rectal tube again in an attempt to get the correct size with minimal air leakage. Had dinner, a fight with Caro and checked Sophie again before bed. All was okay and went back down to our room still very angry with Carolyn. Felt like cancelling Tuesday-night dinner. Tomorrow, I will be going home to either have a swim with Mitchell or play with his slot-car set.

Letter to Sophie, Day 68, Tuesday 24 February 2004
Oh, my beautiful girl, it breaks my heart to see you like this. You are so sick yet you still try to count up to twenty and up to ten and back down again while Matt does physio on you. Your lungs have improved since the weekend. You are on adrenaline for your heart as your blood pressure keeps dropping. I read you stories; you opened your eyes only briefly and squeezed my finger. It seems like the last few weeks have disappeared and we are right back at those first weeks, and I am forever grateful for another day to spend with you. It is a long, hard road, my darling. I saw your spirit again when you were counting with Matt – it was lovely to see. I am very tired but send my energy to you so you can rest and restore. You have a lot of drugs on board to help you through the septic incident. You will have another blood transfusion today.

    We need to move you out of the room on the Burns floor, so I'm just waiting for either Louise or Mum and Dad to arrive so that we can begin the move. I'll bring a lot of stuff upstairs as I want you to feel all the love around you from all the well-wishers you have had in the last two and a half months. I feel it is important to have that spirit around you at this time. Even before we were told of the move, I had brought all your special icons to place them above your head. It is a big battle you face but I want you to win because I know our family will be very, very special. It is already.

Carolyn's journal, Day 68, Tuesday 24 February 2004
A harrowing three days – Sophie became very sick. She was septic and had a team of three doctors and three nurses and the ICU team with her on Saturday morning. She was filled with fluids and taken to PICU. Her central line was changed to a femoral – they tried both groins and the third attempt worked. On the Sunday, Sophie had a rectal tube put in due to poo damaging the graft on her back. They increased the

antibiotics and antifungal drugs, which have potential toxic consequences but there is little choice in the matter. Monday came and she had to be extubated and intubated again. Her tube had a leak from the airways, so they needed to fit a bigger tube – had trouble getting it in, so put the old tube back, then tried the new one again. Her NG tube was out as a result. She had four times the normal dose of muscle relaxants for the procedure. She had a (full) dressing change in the ward this afternoon, as Andy didn't want to take her off the ventilator in the ward. Tonight, she is resting peacefully because she is so sedated.

Ron and I are a mess, shattered that we are back in PICU and that Sophie is so very sick – she doesn't have the strength to sip water through a straw. It is devastating to see her with no energy, as it is her spirit that has really shone through all this. I cradled her in my arms yesterday and it was so sad – her beautiful face all puffy from being prone and from water retention because of the fluid overload. She is still my baby girl and I want her to survive but it looked to me like her fight had gone from her. I do not want her to struggle but I do not want to lose her either.

[Later.] I feel sick – I force myself to eat but feel like throwing up. I am nauseous all the time and I have diarrhoea. My stomach is tight and I feel a tightening all through my chest. I hold my daughter's hand as I pray she pulls through. Andy has called off Thursday's surgery because she is just not well enough. Andy has said we have hit a low. I am so scared. I made myself get out of the unit to sit by her side. My legs are weak and I will them to move down the corridor; my mind can only focus on the most immediate task. Sophie is now on adrenaline. My legs shake and I'm numb; we have to move out of Clubbe Ward. I will not be leaving Sophie's side. I'm almost paralysed with fear. My legs jerk and I itch all over; the same physical symptoms resurface from the first two weeks. I am so tired and emotionally drained.

All I want to do is sleep but I feel guilty for not holding my little girl's hand. Ron is with her and so is Catherine.

Ron's journal, Day 68, Tuesday 24 February 2004
Came up to see Sophie at 7 am, as today I am going home to play with Mitchell and take him to school. Caro went to t'ai chi and I left Sophie sleeping peacefully at 7.30 am. Took Scott to his house and was at my place by 9.10 am. Mitchell and I started putting his slot-car set together. Mitchell then wanted to have a swim; weather not too good but we swam anyway. Mitchell used his flippers and face mask and snorkel. He swam like a fish. Had a great time, then I took Mitchell to school. He took his new toys that he wanted to show his friends. I left him with sadness as usual and went home, always with both the children and Caro in my mind.

I had an 11.30 am meeting with Nadia from OT [occupational therapy] to look at our house to assess its suitability for Sophie. Nadia inspected the house and mentioned that a lift was essential from garage level to the lounge room. We said later the first stop would have to be in the office so that Sophie could go into the middle front garden level and then on to the house (lounge level). Obviously, this would cost a lot more. Next would be the bathroom, which would need to have the shower recess step removed, the floor would have to have non-slip tiles, the privacy screen would have to go, which would mean all the wall tiles would have to be replaced as well. The kitchen would have to have a breakfast servery at Sophie's height; this would mean knocking out a wall, as there is no room for a servery to be fitted. Nadia will have a report ready within the next week or so on the adjustments that would be necessary to meet Sophie's long-term needs.

Back to hospital and Sophie was fairly stable. They were doing physio and getting a lot of spunk out of her. They also started the treatment for the staph infection in the blood. Things seem to be getting worse as time goes on. David and Andy were telling us that the medication is very strong, and that in itself makes the patient sick.

Letter to Sophie, Day 69, Wednesday 25 February 2004
Today, you have done two vomits – enough to put a transpyloric tube in. We wait for an X-ray, more physio and a turn from being prone. It's all a matter of when four nurses are available for the turn. Your lungs are on the mend; your blood pressure varies. Every available corner of the bed has poles and some form of medical equipment attached to monitor everything, ranging from ventilation through to medications. I search for space to put out some hanging crystals, angels and teddies but there is none. I'll have to decorate the walls instead. You are very sedated and I hope this is giving you the rest you need to gain some strength to continue the fight.

People ask if it's hard to see Molly improving so well but I say, 'No, it's wonderful.' I'm just so happy that she's doing so well – it's encouraging and inspiring. We would all like to be there to share the time, but our passage at the moment involves PICU for a little longer than I think everyone expected. I want you to be really well and strong leaving here and am determined to make the next visit to the Burns Unit work better for you. Mitchell's disco was held today and he said, 'Next time, I want Daddy to come and watch Sophie and me dance and sing.'

Carolyn's journal, Day 69, Wednesday 25 February 2004
A calmer day but still I force myself out of bed, force myself to Sophie's room to face what lies ahead. She is still heavily sedated, but things are improving. I picked up Mitchell and then attended his kindy disco. It was strange being amongst normal families again – the children have grown up.

Ron's journal, Day 69, Wednesday 25 February 2004

Woke early and decided to go and see Sophie. She had vomited during the morning and had a temp of 39.3 degrees. Went for some ice to cool her down. A dressing change has been organised today for around 11 am. Andy said he and a Burns nurse will attend. Carrie (nursing-unit manager) came up and apologised for keeping Sophie out of the Burns ward because they are full.

Went back down to the room and started loading the photographs onto CDs. Getting the hang of it. Came back up around 11 am. No Andy, no Burns nurse but we ended up with three nurses from ICU and Jo [Newsome] from physio. Removed about ten more staples and did some physio, and Jo was very happy. I feel the need to get out of the room but feel as though I should stay and be with Sophie.

I wish Caro and I were getting on a little better. We both need each other but with all the stress we hardly say anything nice to each other. I rang the psych doctor yesterday to get an appointment and he said he would get back to me. I need something that can settle me down a bit. I seem to cry a lot at little things that I see. I was driving home last Thursday and stopped at a crossing to see a father and his little child crossing the road. I burst into tears. I feel depressed and need something to get me over it – at least until the worst is over. As I said to Caro a couple of weeks ago, 'My whole life is surrounded by sadness.' Unless I was going through this myself, I couldn't start to realise what it's all about. If I look at or feel Sophie's fingers, I immediately think of her other hand not having fingers, etc., etc.

They have identified Sophie's MRSA and are giving her the appropriate drugs: amphotericin (antifungal), rifampicin, vancomycin.

Letter to Sophie, Day 70, Thursday 26 February 2004

Your chest and lungs have improved and you are down to three chest physios a day. You count and blow bubbles during them. Your rectal tube has blown out three times this evening and you need a blood transfusion. This will stabilise the blood pressure enough to wean you off the adrenaline. So we are making small steps forward. We would love to see you making huge steps forward, but it doesn't work like that and we have learnt after two and a half months just to take each little improvement the days give.

Mitchell is rather over being at hospital, despite lots of activities being on offer. He just needs time in his room to play, so we will try to do that for him tomorrow morning. There is little for him to do in your room except watch a video, which I will arrange as it buys us a little more time and flexibility to be with you or, if you are sleeping, get a picture of your condition and discuss any revision necessary with the doctors. Tomorrow's agenda will be line maintenance and dealing with your vomiting, which you have done twice today; enough so that your jacket needs to be changed – yet more disruption and movement.

A new splint is made for the finger and thumb on your left hand so that they can assume maximum pincer range. This is your daytime splint. You still have night splints for your arms. You are not being placed prone so as not to risk losing your line for your blood pressure, which went into your right leg today. Inaccurate readings have made weaning you off adrenaline difficult – too many bandages and not enough meat on your arms. I love you!

Meet the challenge of change with joy rather than fear.
Anxiety carries a heavy burden, while joy lifts the human spirit.
From *First Aid for a Mother's Soul*

Carolyn's journal, Day 70, Thursday 26 February 2004
Sophie is very heavily sedated but still manages to poo around her rectal tube three times tonight – it has to go! The passage of time seems slow in terms of her recovery. I hope she doesn't stop fighting. Mitchell had Thursday-itis today; I think he is over being at the hospital. We watch the video made for The Journey dinner for Sophie and Molly and cry. All four of us.

Ron's journal, Day 70, Thursday 26 February 2004
Had a few things to do today, starting with an appointment with psych people. Talked about my feelings and about what's going on and how I'm handling it. Ended up with them giving me antidepressant tablets. Not going to tell Caro as she may throw it back in my face. I'm to take one tablet per day. They say it could cause impotence, dizziness and hot flushes, and that it should be taken for at least six months, with meetings every week. We'll see how it goes.

The other job for the day was a meeting with Lincoln Holmes and Cliff Neville from *60 Minutes* in Debra's office [Debra Fowler, public-relations officer at Westmead]. Also invited Allan Martin to attend, to give him input as a family member. He was chuffed. The meeting went well; they said there would probably be about one week of filming and a lot of personal intrusion. We also asked them to connect us with *Women's Weekly* so that *60 Minutes* goes out on the Sunday and *Women's Weekly* comes out on the Monday. We can do radio stuff with Steve Price later. As far as money goes, I was the one to start the conversation by saying any donation will go to the children's trust fund. They will come back to us with a fair offer of a combined amount along with a plan of how it would all work.

Sophie's health has not deteriorated and if anything is getting slightly better. Matt is coming in regularly to do chest physio and is quite happy with how her chest sounds. They decided not to lay Sophie prone tonight so she could rest better. Sophie had another vomit around 11.30 pm. Cleaned her up and left her around 12.30 am for a well-deserved sleep.

Letter to Sophie, Day 71, Friday 27 February 2004
You had an electrocardiogram for your heart and one for your kidneys. You had your eye check for fungus/bacteria. You had a bronchial lavage test for two kinds of bugs. You had your dressings changed. You vomited and pooed around your rectal tube – but we have seen more of the old Sophie sparkling through today. You were playing again with Dad today and tonight you were moving your legs more than I have ever seen you move them. Your lungs are about the same as yesterday. I have some beautiful cards to put on your wall from some schoolchildren in Avalon and heard today via an email from Mum that some schoolchildren in Warkworth [New Zealand] are aware of your accident and how hard you are fighting.

I spoke with Andy today and asked whether, if you had been fully covered with cadaver skin, there would have been less of a chance of you needing to fight so many infections – or whether you might have had more strength to fight infection. I hope that we can donate some funds to research in this field. Your temp is now 39.8, so I do the ice run again. The fan is on and we loosen your dressings. You sleep finally at 7.15 pm, so I hope the many beeps from your monitor don't disturb you – they shouldn't, you must be well used to them by now. I'm re-learning all the readings so I can track your progress. I feel a lot calmer when I sit with you for a few hours.

Carolyn's journal, Day 71, Friday 27 February 2004
It has been a really full-on day. But Sophie wants to move her

legs around more than I have seen before. I spent a chill-out day with Mitchell and he is much calmer. I think I need to do the chill-out day with him every Thursday! It's a strange thing, but Sophie's ventilation sounds like Sophie's breath – her breath that I would listen to when I lay in bed with her when she was having difficulty sleeping before the accident.

Ron's journal, Day 71, Friday 27 February 2004
Woke up late today to a phone call from Greg [Carolyn's brother] in the States. Today is the first day on my tablets; I must admit to being a bit apprehensive about the side effects.

Sophie is up for a number of tests today, starting with a cardiology ultrasound scan. This showed a growth in her heart quite near her valves and the cardiologist said it was probably a bacterial growth that should go away with antibiotics. Next was a kidney scan, which showed no fungal growth at all. Some good news at last.

Rang Rod Smith to email me with a list of things that he needs in the doctor's letter. At around twelve, started feeling a bit nauseous and sick. Was drinking a coffee in Sophie's room and almost vomited. Also feel a bit dizzy, all as they said. I hope it gets better.

Soph also gave blood for culture tests today and had a lung lavage test, which is where they suction samples from well down in her lungs. It's not very pleasant, as they fill her lungs with about 12 ml of saline and will only suck out around 6 ml. Took a couple of times to do it, as the first time they gave her the saline Sophie just coughed it up and vomited. We did it again and it was successful. Today was also a full dressing day. We had nurses Bree and Jill up from Burns, as well as our PICU nurse. Sophie had some ketamine and was fairly comfortable during the whole process. Jo came in and checked some movements – all okay. So today was a big day for Sophie: I hope she sleeps well tonight.

Had dinner donated by an unknown person who knew we liked food from the Himalayan restaurant. Ate dinner in our new courtyard, went up to be with Sophie till around 12.30 am and then off to sleep.

Letter to Sophie, Day 72, Saturday 28 February 2004
You are a little sad today; I long to see you smile but instead the corner of your mouth is turned down. Your transpyloric tube was replaced twice today, so that means X-rays twice. You had two sessions of physio that were shorter than in the past; your third session is tonight. The gastro doctors were reviewing your feeds today and your tummy because of your vomiting. We are again playing catch-up on your feeds.

I sit with you from 10 am until 4 pm, then we look into each other's eyes and you gently close yours. I turn the TV off and you sleep for a bit. You are looking pale, with dark rings under your eyes. It's time to take some more stories, videos and games up to your room, to get you into some more activities. I put some cards on your wall to brighten your room and today a lovely Madeline doll arrives from an anonymous person at the Hopscotch shop in Mosman. She is bigger than you are! I'll bring the *Madeline* video up for you to see.

Molly went home today for a day visit. It was a beautiful sunny day and they had a barbecue together. Our stay in hospital will be a lot longer but I look forward to the day that we can relax at home with you again. I just want to be able to hold you again. Mitchell bought you some bangles today – his choice.

Carolyn's journal, Day 72, Saturday 28 February 2004
Sophie's face is sad today but hopefully she is on the mend. She is being weaned off dopamine and adrenaline and her oxygen too. Ron met Peter Hayward, and if things progress well the

graft could take place next week. But we cannot afford even that much time – we have to achieve full skin coverage as quickly as possible, as the risk of infection and organ failure is so great.

Sophie was harmonised again today. Ron and I admit separately to Caroline and Scott that we thought she was going to die earlier in the week.

Ron's journal, Day 72, Saturday 28 February 2004
Sophie at 39.3 degrees – but the adrenaline is now off. At least we have a positive thing happening. Went for the ice again (I call myself Iceman now). Got her temp down to mid-38s. Andy came in and we went through the records and found no positive culture has been taken since the 25th. Although that's inconclusive, at least it's not negative [i.e. they have not identified an infection being present].

Letter to Sophie, Day 73, Sunday 29 February 2004
Beautiful girl – what a day. Weaned off dopamine and adrenaline. Your TP tube removed and *not* replaced. You were extubated, which left you with a scratchy throat. You had a dressing change and Medazolan withdrawn. The ketamine you had while you had your dressing change, as well as the Medaz reduction, leaves you with an anxious demeanour.

Ron and I sit with you till after 10 pm, when you settle with the help of chloral hydrate. Dad took Mitchell to [his grandson] Oliver's christening; I remember William's, with you looking so beautiful. Lorraine, Fleur and Lee [friends] came to read you stories earlier today. Beth, Allan, Max and Tully [friends] came also. Beth took Mitchell back to Baranbali Avenue afterwards for a picnic lunch. Max brought you a beautiful bear wearing a pink tutu. Trudy and [son] Zach came tonight.

Everyone wants you to get better soon, as everyone misses you so very much. My precious little.

Carolyn's journal, Day 73, Sunday 29 February 2004
What a huge day. No feeds since 6 am in anticipation of the extubation. Gemma will grade her NG feeds up overnight but huge catch-up will need to be played. Sophie shows signs of ketamine shock: hallucinations much like the startle reflex in babies. She scares easily with any noise, her legs and arms flay, she looks around anxiously. A larger tube was required when they had problems intubating her. It grazed her throat, so coughing is difficult and painful for her. Sophie slept one hour in twenty-four and is very overtired – wired, I call it – so we will give her chloral hydrate to settle her. She may also have diazepam if necessary – she needs a good night's rest to sleep off all the side effects of the drugs. She startles every five minutes for over an hour.

Letter to Sophie, Day 74, Monday 1 March 2004
Starts with a big vomit at 5 am; you have not slept much in the last forty-eight hours. Your eyes roll back in your head, you sweat, you are anxious and your blood pressure rises. Your body twitches; it is less obvious than yesterday, but it is still very worrying. This morning, you have been blowing bubbles with Matt and Beckie; you also showed them how you played the recorder and harmonica. You blew more bubbles with Gemma tonight. We had lots of conversations with doctors and doctors' teams today.

It is lovely to see you smile and lovely to hear your voice. I wish that you could have just one peaceful, event-free day. PICU have assured me that you will not be leaving the ward till you are one hundred per cent ready to go to the Burns Unit.

Peter Hayward says he wants to make sure you are really well and back on the Burns ward before you have your head grafted. I can't wait for the day you are fully grafted. x

Carolyn's journal, Day 74, Monday 1 March 2004
Arrive at Sophie's room to find bubbles have been blown after physio with Matt – Beckie was on and encouraged her also. Stories in between doctors' chats, which are endless. Feeds recommenced and back up to 40 ml by 7 pm. Sophie is either fitting or on Medaz withdrawals. I stay with her till 10 pm; I will not leave her without a nurse. I head back up to her bed again at 11 pm to lie with her and comfort her.

Ron's journal, Day 74, Monday 1 March 2004
Gemma rang at twelve, saying that Sophie wanted me. Went up there to find Sophie wide awake and still going through shocks. We ended up giving her Valium to calm her down and she finally went to sleep at 2.30 am. Came up later in the morning and spoke to Scott again, who said that Molly went through the same thing and it went into the next day before it settled down. Ended up speaking to Dr David. David went through all of the medication that Sophie is on and said that all the symptoms that Sophie has – vomiting, diarrhoea, scared, startled, eyes rolling – could be from withdrawal, as Medazolan was normally given by IV drip continuously for only four days. Sophie has been on it for eight days and then went cold turkey.

I felt very sick today. All of the things the psych doctor said – nausea, increased urination, dizziness, the lot. Caro spent most of the time with Soph today.

Spoke to Trudy a number of times today. *60 Minutes* came back with an offer for both *60 Minutes* and *Woman's Day*. Trudy told me and I said forget it. She also spoke to Lincoln, who said they would come back with a counter offer; he came back and said we either accept that offer or forget about everything. We will see what happens.

Sophie looks so beautiful just lying there at 11 pm. She needs to rest so much. Please don't wake. 11.10 pm checked her temperature and she was 39.4 degrees. Mr Iceman in action again and the ibuprofen.

chapter seven
withdrawal

Sophie continues to suffer symptoms of withdrawal from the sedative that she has been on for eight days. Ron and Carolyn can only watch – even reinstating the drug would do nothing to counteract these symptoms, as the reaction simply needs to run its course.

For Sophie's friend and fellow patient Molly, it is time to go home. Ron and Carolyn delight in her progress and dream of the day when they, too, can be home as a family again.

Letter to Sophie, Day 75, Tuesday 2 March 2004
I read you stories in the morning. You have your dressing change at 2 pm and all I want for you is a quiet, restful day. An electrocardiogram is scheduled for the morning but in fact doesn't happen at all – it's put off till tomorrow due to priorities. They just want to check the clot in your heart to make sure we can proceed with surgery. Unfortunately, you have a bad reaction to the drugs needed for the bath and you are terribly agitated in

the evening. You are totally overtired, having had about ten hours' sleep in the last seventy-two, then your eyes start to roll back in your head. We hadn't seen this since Monday about 8 pm. We take your plaster cast off because we don't want you to hurt your tummy; you repeatedly hit it and yell. It is dreadful to watch. I leave at 3 am, after you have finally settled. I look at you sleeping so peacefully now and pray that God will let you have some peace and rest. You have the most beautiful serene face, my little angel, considering all that you endure.

Letter to Sophie, Day 76, Wednesday 3 March 2004

Molly went home today. What a joyous day for them, yet we will miss them all so much – our dinner parties for the last three months. Mitchell cried when he saw the TV coverage of Lilly and Molly going.

Your clonidine has been increased and your morphine increased to sedate you. You sleep a lot. I've asked if Bettina can keep your door closed so as not to interrupt your rest. Daddy spends time with you in the afternoon when you wake, with Grandma and Grandpa visiting, Catherine and John as well. You are much more settled. Paul brings you some books – stories work well at the moment, as you are not awake enough to engage in much else. We want you calm and rested, so the blinds are down.

I head home to pick up Mitchell, having aired our theories on pain with the pain fellow and on dressings with Carrie – we have made some adjustments for tomorrow's dressing change.

When Scott made a press statement on leaving the hospital with Molly, he made a lovely comment about the job not being done until Sophie is home. We have been very lucky to share the experience with them. They are and will remain very special friends.

Carolyn's journal, Day 76, Wednesday 3 March 2004
The last forty-eight hours have been a horror of trying to establish what is wrong with Sophie; it appears she has been suffering drug withdrawals, coupled with her lack of sleep. We are waiting for her electrocardiogram to see if her heart is able to sustain the graft, which, if given the okay by ICU, will be Thursday or Friday. Today, having been completely knocked out by clonidine, she slept, making up for the severe deprivation of the last seventy-two hours. Yesterday, her eyes were rolling again; she started hitting herself with her hand for hours, yelling and generally in a high state of distress. This morning was much the same, although she had had four hours' sleep. I didn't enter her room today till 10 pm. I stood outside this morning and afternoon but was very fearful that my presence would wake her. She had clearly been distressed by movement, sound, people – I think she is suffering from sensory overload. It was devastating to see.

Letter to Sophie, Day 77, Thursday 4 March 2004
A better day again – in fact, I could say a good day. You had a dressing change. We used a different dressing. You are more settled and, with regular clonidine, you are getting more regular blocks of sleep. You liked some stories and we used the felt board in the evening, which you enjoyed as your story time before going to sleep. We have a new calming sleep oil for your pillow, which includes lavender and camomile. We have soothing music and you are asleep at 9 pm. It feels like a rested day for everyone.

Caroline rang this evening to see how we were doing. She said their first day at home was a bit stressful. Scott was speaking at the golf function on behalf of both families. So many people have arranged functions for fund-raising and so many have put in a huge effort to assist, it has been amazing. Debra Fowler spoke to me today and told me it has been her biggest story in her fourteen years at the hospital. We feel humbled by the effort of the hospital and the wider community, and it's all because they think you are a very, very special girl. You ate minestrone soup tonight!

Letter to Sophie, Day 78, Friday 5 March 2004
Today, you are scheduled for a new central line and grafts. You have been fasted since 4 am; we were originally scheduled for 11 am but it was not to be. You had IV fluids and a small amount of water and milk at eleven, because you were desperate for water and ice. David Murrell, Gemma and Jonathan [Gillis, ICU specialist] all went in to bat for you to be prioritised. You were on the emergency list and there were fifteen cases. That adds to the busy theatre day the hospital already has. Usually, Tuesday and Thursday are the Burns theatre days, so that is why we are on the emergency list. We are learning the protocol of hospital life and its politics. One thing is very clear: they could do with a lot more funding, despite the good work they do.

Your graft went well, although your head is not fully covered. Peter Hayward has left the back of the head to complete along with your back and bottom – another op when you will go prone afterwards. Peter comments on how much morphine it takes to sedate you. It has been nearly three months. You will be X-rayed to check your line – Amy is on tonight, so you are in good hands.

Carolyn's journal, Day 78, Friday 5 March 2004
The last forty-eight hours have been better for Sophie; she is more rested because of the six-hourly clonidine. She engages in stories and felt boards and is easier to settle. We are advised she

is growing more bugs from her femoral line, which was replaced during the week. They pre-empted this by placing her on more antibiotics. The one for her heart will need to run for six weeks through her central line. Today, a new central surgical line was fitted, and I pray that this lasts and does not get infected – she needs some wins on her side for a change.

Letter to Sophie, Day 79, Saturday 6 March 2004
A calm day. Your NG tube was changed; other than that, you were largely left alone. You were very sleepy, had a good four hours' sleep last night and two and a half hours late afternoon. You are behind in your feeds and Peter Hayward wants to give you extra protein shakes to fatten you up. He wants your skin and donor site to heal. Dave and Louise visit, and Lee and Linda; Katrina came to help look after Mitchell. Catherine brought Nana and Nanu to see you. You closed your eyes when they came in the room – a little shy, Nana said. They were very pleased to see you.

Peter is very pleased with how your legs and arms are healing, and we are hoping to reduce your medications during your dressing change because they are doing so well. Gemma has been looking after you again today. It's lovely having a nurse who knows you so well and can assist in formulating a plan for the day or use her judgement to make recommendations for a change to your regime. All the Burns ward nurses ask after you and are looking forward to having you back on the ward. I am so proud of you, my beautiful girl.

Carolyn's journal, Day 79, Saturday 6 March 2004
A peaceful day. We lobbied with Peter Hayward to postpone Sophie's dressing change till Sunday morning. It seems the first day that Sophie has had so little done to her for months. I feel

withdrawal

that she is really rested and can start coming off the clonidine so she is more awake during the day. It is difficult to engage Sophie in anything more than stories and the odd whistle blow while she is so sedated. It looks like we will be close to getting to the Burns ward again early next week, with another graft for patch-ups during the week. Peter doesn't want to lose momentum.

Letter to Sophie, Day 80, Sunday 7 March 2004
Twelve weeks today. David and Janet [Binks, friends], Beth, Trudy and Zach, Mandy and Margaret [Henry] came to visit today. They shared in reading you stories. Mandy brought you beautiful bandannas with bangles to match. Mitchell keeps asking, 'When will Sophie be better like Molly?' and we say that one day we will be going home like Molly and Lilly. We look forward to that day so much. We have been told we have Molly's old room in the Burns ward and I hope to be there tomorrow.

Carolyn's journal, Day 80, Sunday 7 March 2004
I left at midnight and Sophie woke on and off throughout the night. She did a vomit in the early hours of Sunday morning but had a better day generally, with a few more smiles and a big cuddle with Dad after the dressing change. Mitchell stood on the chair next to Sophie's bed to say, 'I love you, Sophie,' and I could see the fear in his eyes. He left to go home and I miss him already.

Letter to Sophie, Day 81, Monday 8 March 2004
What an exciting day – back on the Burns ward and back to your old room! [A change of circumstances meant that Sophie was given her own old room, rather than Molly's.] I've started

decorating it already. You have been in a happy, chatty, cheeky mood. Gemma said, 'Just like the Sophie of old!' You played hide-and-seek peek-a-boo with Martin, the nurse in the room next door, and giggled spontaneously for the first time since being in hospital. I held you today, which was beautiful, and you sat in your chair for over an hour chatting to the many visitors that came in to see you on your last day in PICU, hopefully for a long time!

I changed your nappy today. Because you have pooed three rectal tubes out, we have gone back to nappies for a while. We are back into the very hands-on approach in the Burns ward and this time round I'm determined to make it work. You will have a GP overseeing your case. Although you did a big vomit, you seem to be tolerating your feeds and ate a little sandwich for lunch and a tiny amount for dinner. A large request list through the day, though: meat, sausage, bone, ham – at least there is some interest there! I'll try to vary the diet over the next week or so with some yummy treats.

You finally settle tonight with a slightly earlier dose of chloral and clonidine; Dad and I ate in your room. You seem to settle more easily in the ward environment than you do at PICU. This apparently is not unusual and it is because in PICU patients don't distinguish between night and day. And so we embark on phase two of your healing – three months down the track!

Carolyn's journal, Day 81, Monday 8 March 2004
Sophie moved! And I feel a lot more confident this time around. I've even changed a nappy on my own. Sophie was in good spirits today but has had little sleep the last two nights, so here's hoping she has a settled night tonight – I'm on duty. A new pain regime is being discussed and another new drug considered for pain and sleep. I really, really want to go home and I miss Mitchell.

Letter to Sophie, Day 82, Tuesday 9 March 2004

A blood transfusion and a chest X-ray are required today. You have little sleep at quiet time due to interruptions. Grandma Joy stays reading to you; she is off to New Zealand for ten days and a walk in Akaroa (Banks Peninsula). I hope Dad will be okay with Mitchell next week, although I have Dot [volunteer] coming over to help out in the evenings. We got you in your seat today and you seem happy about that, although you complain that your back hurts. It's great to see you sitting up again. We are reviewing the splint regime as well as the physio regime. Although you find it uncomfortable lying on your side, you roll back on your own and we clap and say, 'Sophie can roll – wee!' And you say, 'Weeee,' as well – it is just priceless. You are practising your yoga when we do nappy changes and are so proud, saying, 'I do yoga. I do yoga.' Daddy slept with you tonight but by all accounts not much sleep was to be had.

Ron's journal, Day 82, Tuesday 9 March 2004

Went to Sophie's room at 7.15 am to pick up some tax papers for Caro and me to take home. Sophie has had a good night's sleep and was very peaceful when I arrived. The traffic going home was enormous as there was an accident on the M2 freeway, so it took around an hour and a half to get home. I was greeted by a great reception from Mitchell, who is always happy to see me. We played for a while and I drew him a dinosaur, which I cut out for him to take to school. Worked till around twelve and then back to the hospital. Sophie was doing well today, with her vital signs good except for her respiratory rate at around sixty per minute – it should be down around forty per minute. Peter came in and had a chat about tomorrow's operation and said we would take skin from another place on her body so that they can cover what they can.

Letter to Sophie, Day 83, Wednesday 10 March 2004
It's 10 pm and I'm off in search of ham; it's just as well Lyn, your ward granny, brought some in for you at lunchtime. She sits with you Monday, Wednesday and Friday for a few hours to keep you company while you sleep, and we have meetings, pick up Mitchell, go to work or attend to domestic duties. Today, Captain Starlight visited and sang you 'Old MacDonald', 'Twinkle Twinkle' and 'In the Jungle'. Geata, Laura and Amanda visited with a gift from a Dick Smith employee – your own DVD and TV (paid for out of his own pocket). People have been so generous and their daily support helps us to help you to get well.

Today, you sit in your chair and move both hands to the storyboard on your table. You use your fingers to move pieces around and dress a puzzle of a little girl. You did really well. Today was another treat for me. I had a big hug with you as you sat on my lap facing outwards. It was beautiful feeling your body on mine. We spent forty-five minutes like that. I feel a sense of calm today as I see your progress, and although you were fasted till 3 pm because you were possibly going to have surgery, you seemed pleased to do things. Catherine visited, as did John and Kate and Lee. Grandpa brought Mitchell to hospital, so you had a busy day with little sleep because of interruptions to your room and phone calls – you still startle easily.

Carolyn's journal, Day 83, Wednesday 10 March 2004
Two days in the ward and we are slowly establishing a routine. It is clear, however, that constant interruptions are a disturbance, so we will try to manage these through limiting access to Sophie's room. Sophie had a blood transfusion yesterday. Her loss of potassium is still an issue and albumin is required all the time. There is continued monitoring of Sophie's fluid intake in combination with drugs, antibiotics and feeds. Sophie is not tolerating additional drinks other than water. Ron did not have a restful night with her last night due to constant interruptions

and beeping monitors. I will address this in an attempt to improve sleeping patterns.

I had to postpone my meetings because of impending surgery. They will have to happen next week. I've tried to get to work the last two Wednesdays but unscheduled things happen with Sophie and it proved too difficult.

Ron's journal, Day 83, Wednesday 10 March 2004
Not a very good sleep at all. Up most of the night for a number of reasons. It's amazing how they expect kids to sleep when they have all the pump alarms turning on, all at different times. The nurses come in and reset one alarm, knowing that another alarm will go off in five minutes, and so on. Sophie has five pumps putting morphine or antibiotics or blood into her, so the alarms are continuous. The other thing that keeps Sophie awake is plain pain. She often wakes with twitches of pain, so there is a continuous reassuring that goes on all night. Then there's the fixation with water. She would keep on drinking water all day if we let her. But if she has too much, she vomits, so we have to say 'no' and change her thoughts to something else. Then there's nappy changes. Sophie seems to dirty her nappy about six times a day. Each nappy change and dressing clean-up takes about half an hour, and it can't wait due to the risk of infection to graft sites, bare sites or donor sites. Overall, there are plenty of reasons for Sophie not to sleep. Sophie even woke up last night telling me she was upside down. The ritual now is to tell her that you have just turned her back again.

Sophie was pretty quiet today; I think she is just too tired. She was to have another skin graft today. Peter was doing a major operation, with three medical teams from cardiology finishing up with Peter's team. Peter was going to let us know around twelve that if the operation was too big they would have to postpone Sophie's operation till tomorrow. We got the message around 3 pm that our operation was cancelled.

Scott and Caroline, Lilly and Molly came over today for Molly's physio and our meeting with Trudy and Debra Fowler about *60 Minutes* and other show offers. We all agreed in principle that we would go with *60 Minutes* with some provisions. We then had lunch together and talked about life on the outside. Allan brought Mitchell over about 5.30 pm and seemed very tired. Caro's turn to sleep with Soph tonight and me with Mitchell. John and Kate came over for a visit before we retired for the night. Sleep well, Sophie and Caro.

Letter to Sophie, Day 84, Thursday 11 March 2004
My brave little girl, you had surgery again today – two small grafts on your leg and hand. You needed your NG tube replaced and your paediatrician is looking into potassium loss, which may have an impact on your kidneys. You sat and played with your toys at the table, then slept for about an hour and a half in your chair.

Post-op, you are a little agitated. Linda comes to visit and gives you water to drink. Dad gets your TV and DVD going, so you watch DVDs with Mitchell. You keep calling his name and he holds your hand. He has invented a 'lesson' about magic coming from the water drunk by dinosaurs going into their bones and sending magic to all the sick children – Ben, Molly, Sophie and all the others. You slept in blocks of two hours and were quite awake, making demands between 2 and 5 am. You are very imaginative, particularly when it comes to food – pizza was what you wanted. Your knees hurt, you were thirsty and just generally restless. I'll get you up sitting on my knee again tomorrow and focus on some instrument playing. Lisa, the play therapist, brought you some more things to play with and was very pleased to see you moving your arms so well. You ate soup and ham for dinner.

withdrawal

Carolyn's journal, Day 84, Thursday 11 March 2004
A small graft today on hand and leg. Sophie was restless in recovery; lots of water demanded and, once back in her room, it was all vomited up. Sophie watched *Spirit* the movie on TV and, as a train chased the horse down the hill, she said to Dad, 'I dead, I dead.' Mitchell had a session with Sandra, as did Ron – Sandra said Mitchell has raised some interesting things, but I've yet to find out what issues were discussed.

A sleepless night with Sophie leaves you pretty thin on the ground resource-wise. I had about four hours and it wears you out emotionally. I found her post-op withdrawals difficult to deal with and the irrational demands very draining. Sophie blew her cheeks out at me last night, went bright red and groaned a guttural growl: 'I eat you, I eat you.' She keeps repeating intermittently, 'Help me, help me, I scared.' Today, she was red in the face again and growling like a tiger. Mitchell came to say goodnight to her and she just kept repeating his name. I told him it was because she loved him. He gently held her bandaged hand and said 'yes, Sophie, yes, Sophie' – a poignant moment in a shattered family life.

Ron's journal, Day 84, Thursday 11 March 2004
Played the new *Lion King* video for Mitchell before heading off for breakfast. The biomedical department picked up the new TV and DVD for testing before returning them to our room. Sophie is going to get more skin grafts today. Peter Hayward wants to keep the momentum going, even if it means doing patchwork on Sophie. He is keen not to lose any time. Sophie's temp has seemed to stabilise a lot lately; ever since she has been on the correct antibiotics for her staph infection, she has not been over thirty-nine degrees. When she gets to 38.5, we give her paracetamol and it settles down.

Caro is in a grumpy mood today. Lack of sleep is what I put it down to. Picked Mitchell up from Sandra. She says he is such a good boy but he has a few issues that we need to discuss. One is that he thinks Sophie's limbs will grow back by themselves. We will meet with Sandra later to follow this up.

Sophie is called up to theatre and we went through the routine we have gone through so many times before: wheeling her up to the theatre, pressing the button to open the automatic doors and go to the waiting area, where the anaesthetist has a talk to us to check the authorisation form, etc. I get dressed up in my gown, hair net and shoe covers. Caro says goodbye to Sophie as she is wheeled away to go into theatre and I hold her hand and go with her. I keep on asking Soph if she is a big, strong girl, getting her to repeat it as we go. I then tell her that Mum can't hear her and that she needs to say it louder and louder until she is yelling it out. We get into the theatre foyer, where they prepare Sophie for the anaesthetic. I always ask the doctor to let me know when he is going to give her the drugs to make her sleep so I can give her a kiss and tell her I love her before she goes under. When she goes to sleep, I then cry and walk back out to the waiting room to de-robe and meet up with Caro.

This time, had some coffee with Linda and waited. It's not only the present operation that is my worry; it's what they find of the last skin graft that is a problem. We got a call at 3.30 to say she was out of the operation. Spoke to Andy in recovery, who told us that Sophie's last head skin graft only took to thirty per cent of her head, so we lost seventy per cent of the graft. In this case, one step forward, two steps back. But he did say that all of her other areas are healing well.

Sophie seems in a lot of pain after this operation. Went back to her room and got settled in. It was my turn to take care of Sophie tonight. The first problem came when she did a poo. Firstly, there was no nappy and secondly there was no rectal tube like we had asked. Thirdly, because of the rectal tube not being there, the poo was everywhere. Unfortunately, they had used skin from her bottom as a donor site (as well as other sites) and had grafted the top of her left leg and covered these areas with a stapled-on covering. Some of this covering was already soiled and no one knew what had been done and how to deal with it. We all did our best in cleaning it up. Only one or two hours' sleep the whole night. It was an absolutely awful night.

Letter to Sophie, Day 85, Friday 12 March 2004

It's a tough day today. You didn't sleep well last night with Dad and he really feels the effect. Mitchell is tired as well, but fortunately Mary comes and he goes to sleep at 6.30 pm. We really need to establish a sleep cycle with you, both for midday and at night. Your pain medication is under review and oral morphine is suggested, with diazepam being reduced. You have a familiar pattern when you don't want to go to sleep: first you say you want more food, then you say 'my knee is sore'.

We have changed your nasal prongs to infant size. They continually rubbed an area of your nose, but the smaller ones are much better – one less irritating thing for you and me. I put your lullabies on because it's 9 pm and still you are not asleep. You drift off but startle easily when the nurses come close to your bed.

Carolyn's journal, Day 85, Friday 12 March 2004

A stressful day. I'm concerned at Sophie's agitation and asked some teams to talk about her outside. Ron disagrees and then we argue. He's had a really bad night with Sophie and the day turns to shit. He's stressed, I got stressed because of him and then we have Mitchell to deal with as well. I'm of the opinion that we need to get Ron home and Mitchell in day care for an additional day. It is tough trying to be present for him as well and one less day means one less day of pressure. We will need to discuss this with Sandra to make sure she is still able to meet with him weekly and with Ron and myself. I can stay Sunday to Thursday on my own, sleep when Sophie does and somehow create a better sleeping pattern for her. I found today very difficult – it's not often I need paracetamol.

Sophie vomits her meds because she doesn't like the change of sensation from her NG tube. It's almost a deliberate action.

Another day on the battlefield – enemies from every side. Every ten minutes, another alarm goes off just when you settle, so you wake. It's chronic sleep deprivation.

Ron's journal, Day 85, Friday 12 March 2004
Woke up really exhausted and sick from the lack of sleep. The pain team came in and Caro asked them not to discuss matters at Sophie's bedside. I had an argument about this and walked off with the shits and went back to the unit with Mitchell. I went to sleep for around an hour and a half or two hours, as I was exhausted and felt sick. This was the first time in three months here that I have had a sleep in the afternoon. Mark and Lee came over and took Mitchell and Caro to Westfield to buy some extras for Mitchell's fish tank, while I took care of Sophie. When they came back, I went and had a couple of hours with Mark and Lee and Mary, then some dinner. I didn't get through the full dinner as I started to vomit. I was out for the count for the night.

chapter eight
turning the corner

Increasingly, the peaks and troughs of the Delezios' emotional roller coaster become evident, with blissful days flanked by bleak ones. Sleep – or lack of it – is all-important. For Sophie, it is a mark of her recovery, while for her parents a full night's sleep is a dimly remembered dream.

Ron and Carolyn try to keep their perspective and maintain a semblance of calm by looking forward to the rehab phase of Sophie's care: the stage when they will be helping Sophie to move, to play and to learn, rather than engaging in the elemental battle for survival that has been their lives for three months now.

Letter to Sophie, Day 86, Saturday 13 March 2004
A calm, happy day. Daddy, Mitchell, you and I watched *Babe* this morning and you sat on my knee. This afternoon, Dad was telling Catherine directions and mentioned McDonald's. You said, 'I want go McDonald's too.' So Catherine brought you

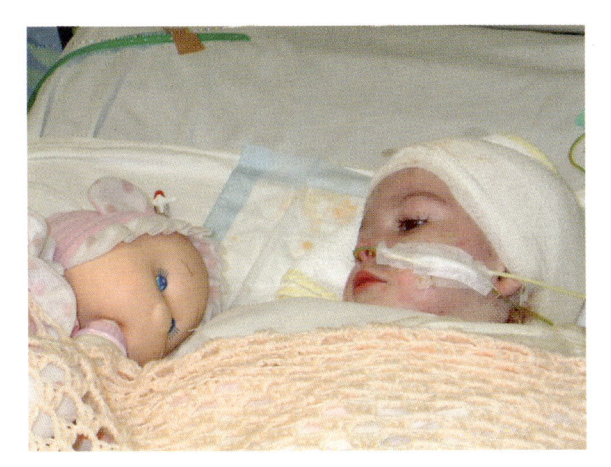

February 2004: Unable to move for long periods of time, Sophie would lie in her hospital bed and watch. She knew everything that was going on in the room.

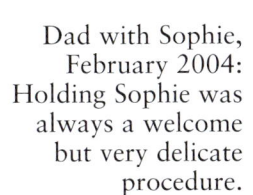

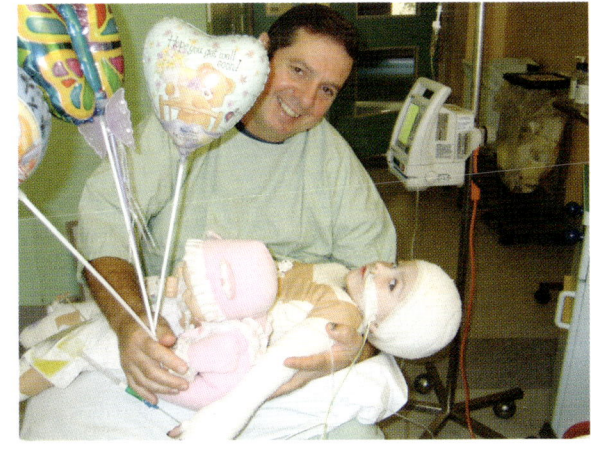

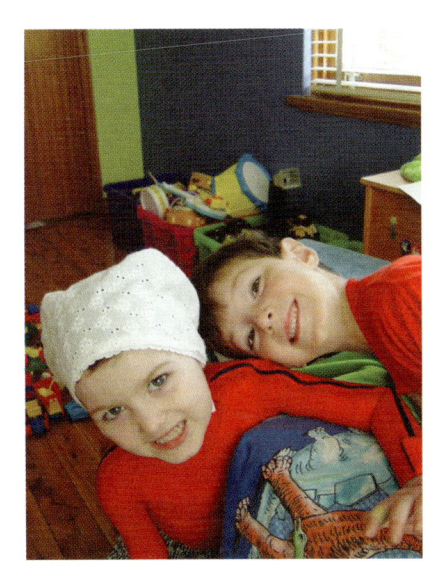

Dad with Sophie, February 2004: Holding Sophie was always a welcome but very delicate procedure.

Mitchell with Sophie, April 2005: 'My big brother, Mitchell, is the best!'

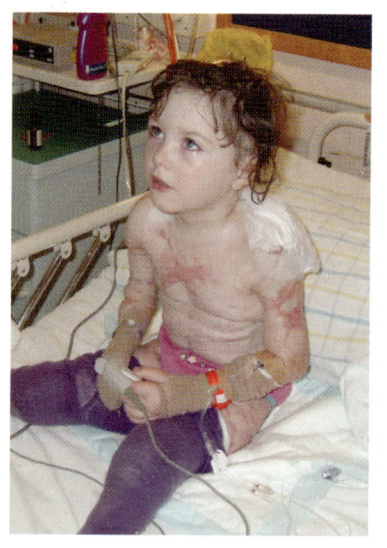

Sophie watching TV, July 2005: 'No! I want to watch Captain Starlight!'

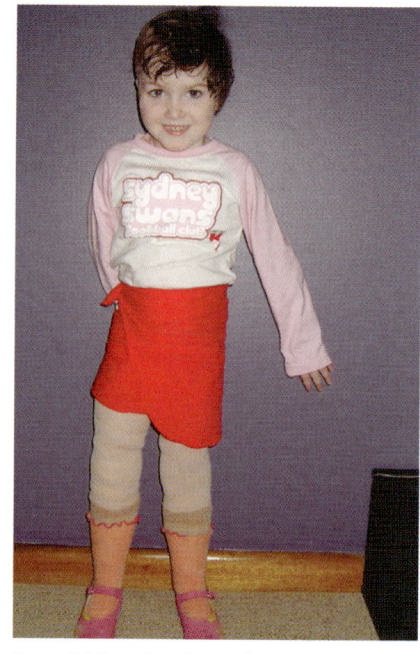

July 2005: Sophie, the Sydney Swans fan, wearing her prosthetic legs.

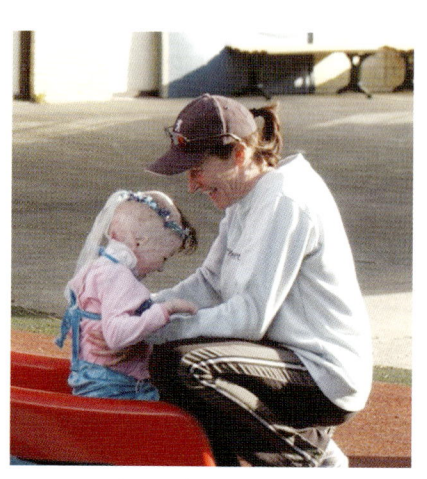

Mum with Sophie, August 2005: Sophie achieved a lot at Arranounbai School. She loved to slide – the faster the better.

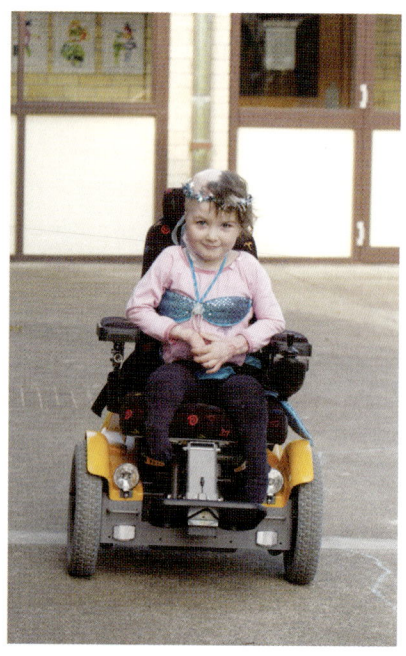

Sophie's new wheelchair, August 2005: 'I can climb into it myself.'

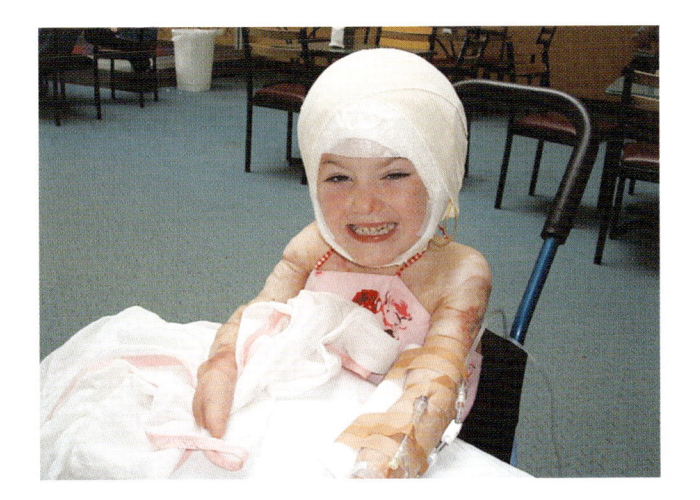

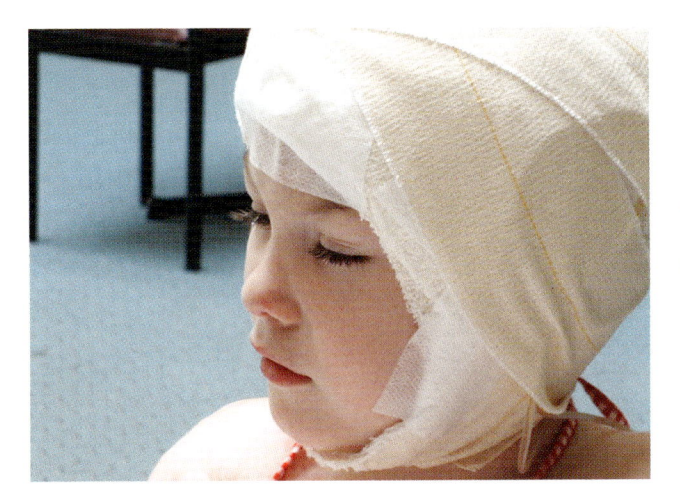

October 2005: Sophie after her first hair operation.

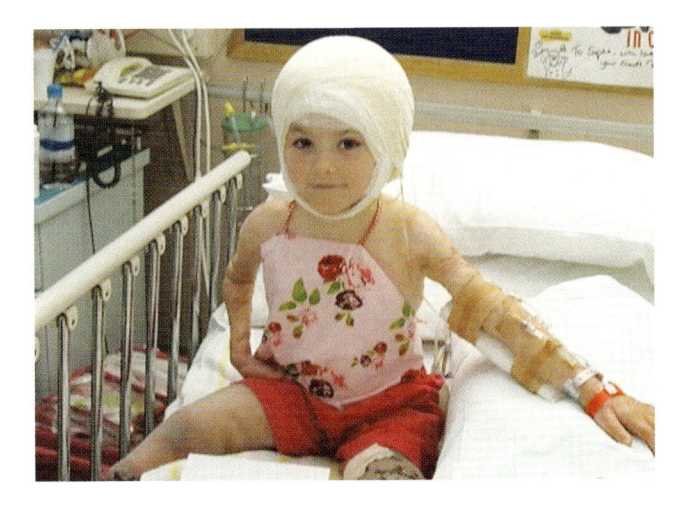

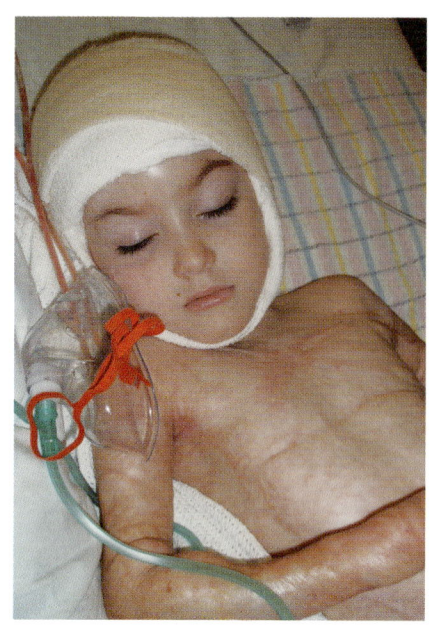

October 2005: Sophie never liked the oxygen mask on her face. The closest we could get it was to her side and usually only when she slept.

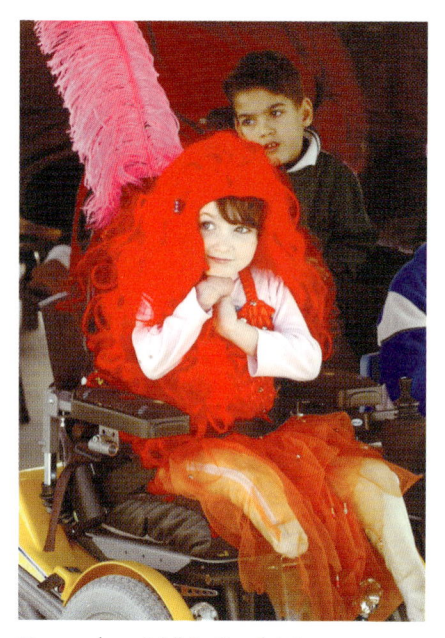

December 2005: Sophie's farewell party at Arranounbai School.

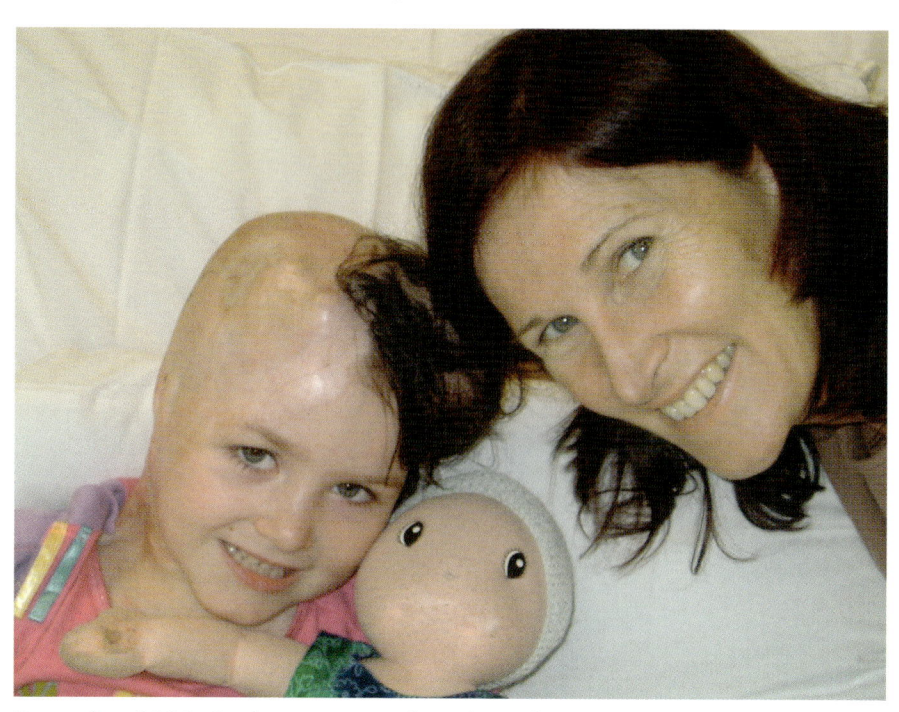

December 2005: Sophie, Mum and Sophie's favourite doll, Mags, in hospital.

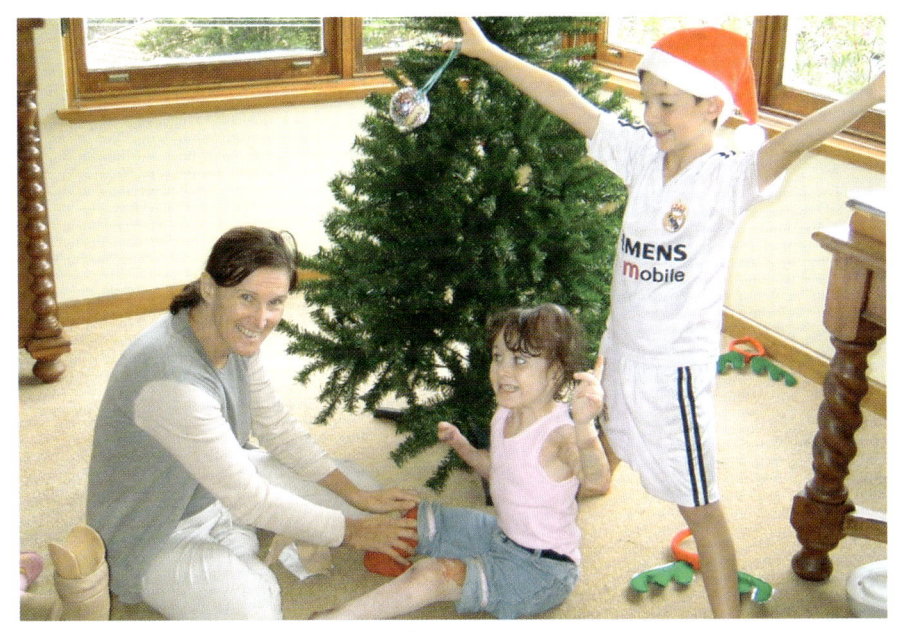

Getting ready for Christmas in 2005 – always an exciting time.

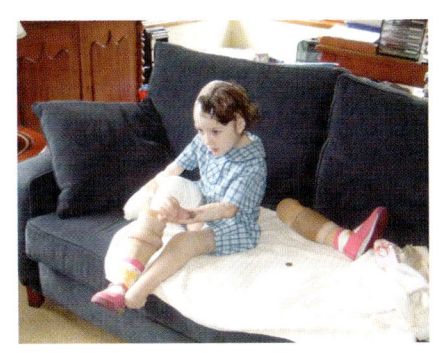

January 2006: Practising for school.

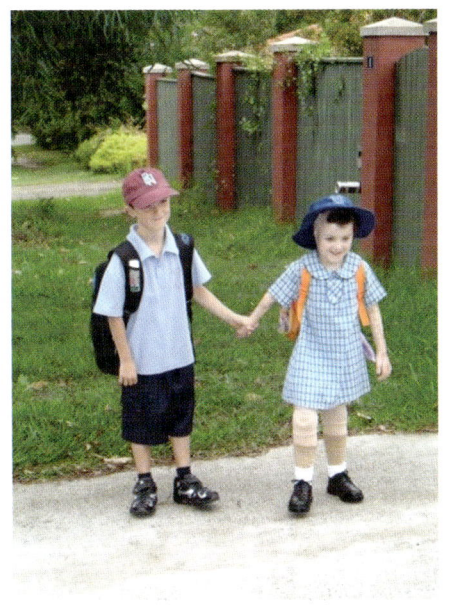

January 2006: Mitchell accompanying Sophie on her first day at school.

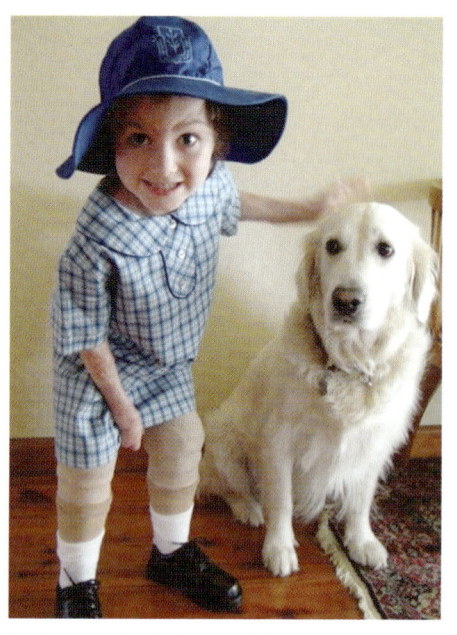

February 2006: 'And this is my assistance dog, Tara.'

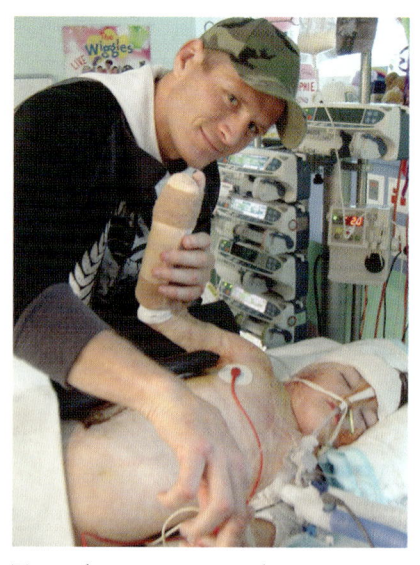

Two champions together, May 2006: The incredible moment when Sophie, still in a coma after her second accident, raised her hand for Danny Green.

May 2006: Sophie moving from Intensive Care in Sydney Children's Hospital at Randwick and feeling pretty happy about it.

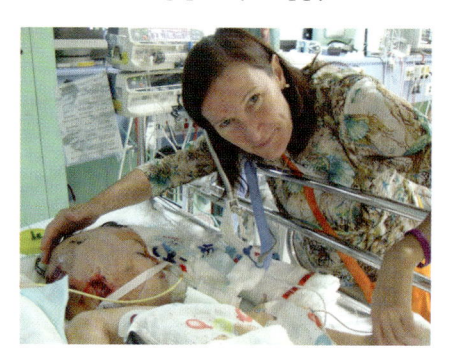

May 2006: Every day, Sophie gets a little bit stronger.

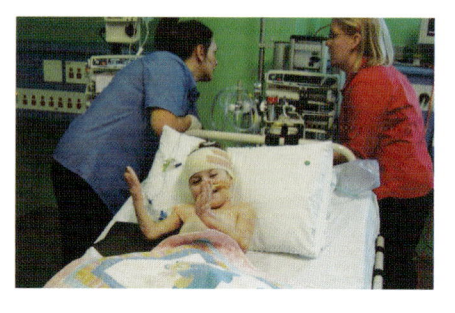

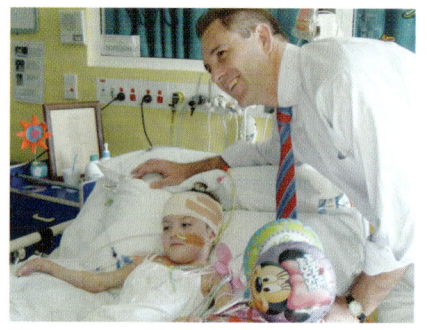

May 2006: Dr Jonny Taitz treated Sophie following both her accidents.

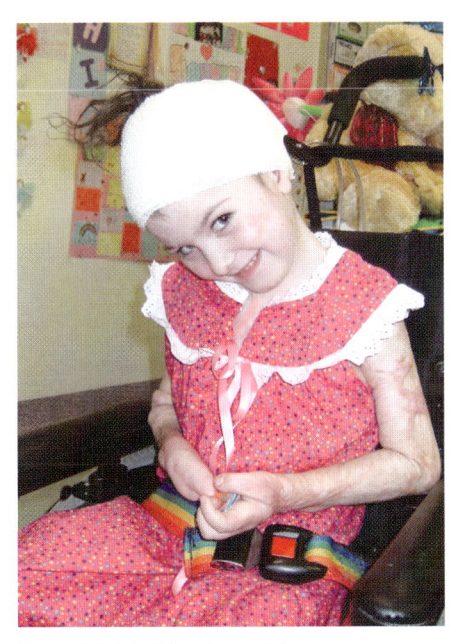

June 2006: The 'can I have a packet of chips, please' look.

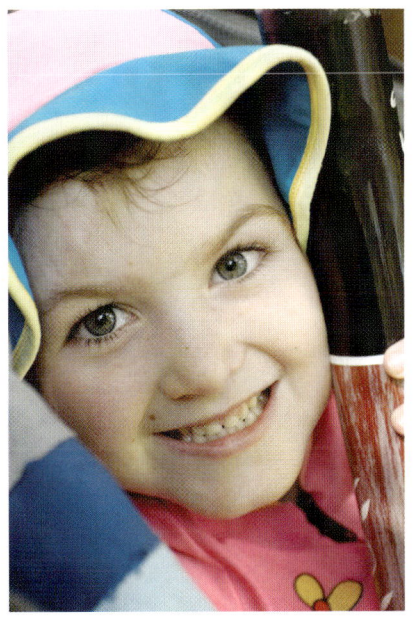

September 2006: 'Me and my didgeridoo.' (© New Idea/Paul Broben)

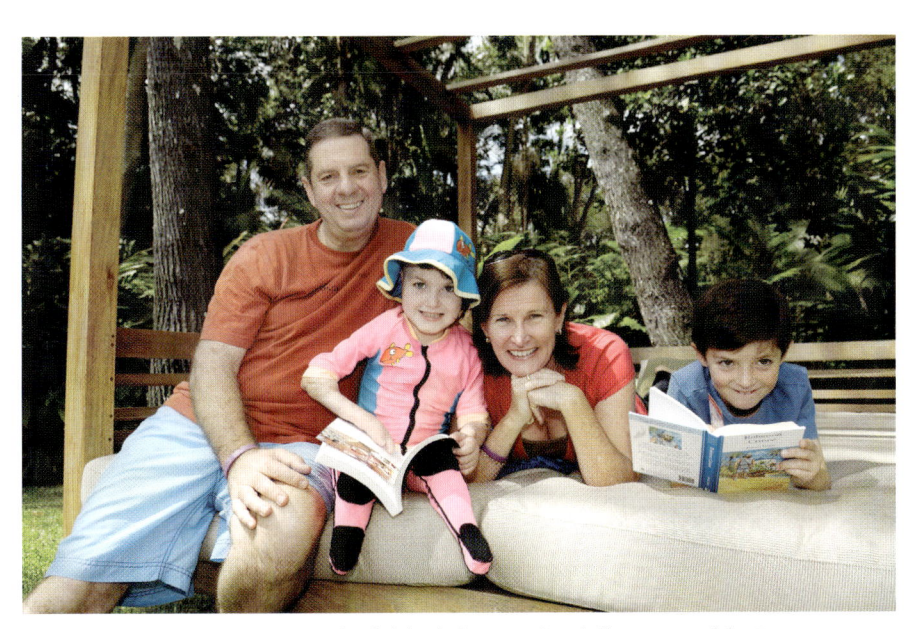

September 2006: Our wonderful holiday at the fully accessible Byron at Byron Resort and Spa. Many thanks to our fantastic hosts, Lyn and John Parche. (© New Idea/Paul Broben)

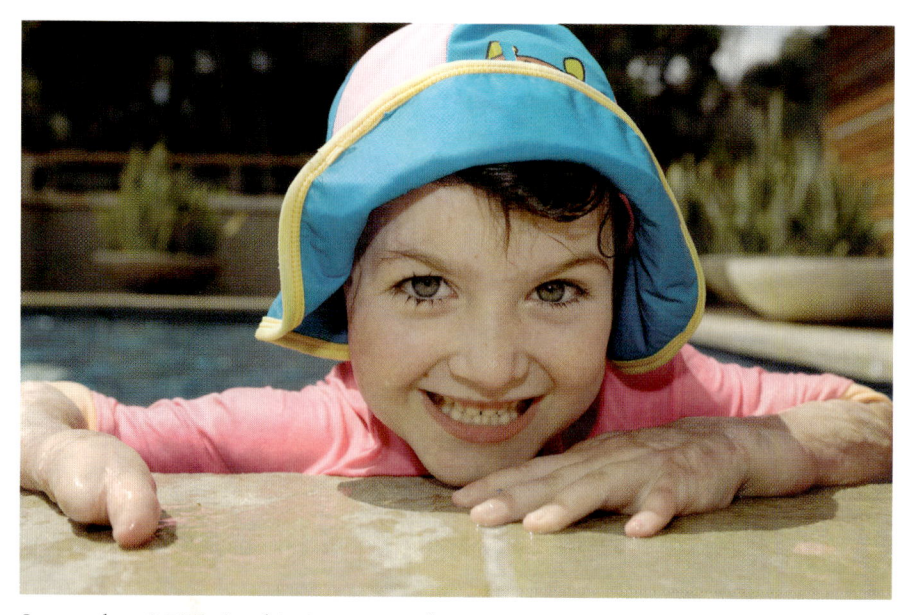

September 2006: Sophie is a natural swimmer. (© New Idea/Paul Broben)

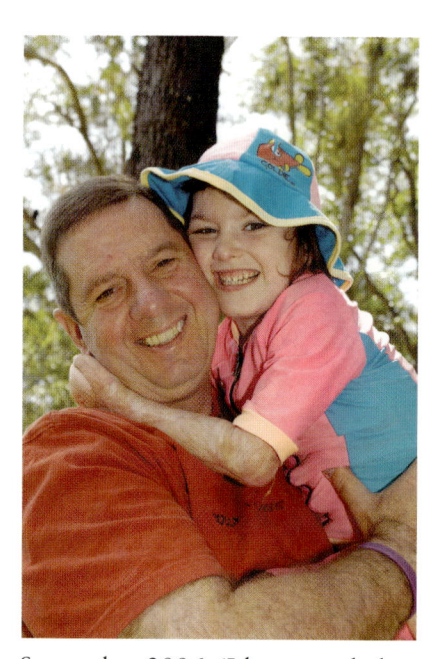

September 2006: 'I love my dad. He is very funny.' (© New Idea/Paul Broben)

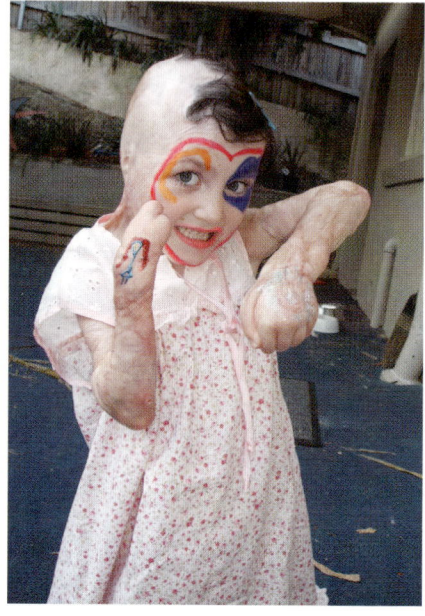

October 2006: Sophie at home, doing the Danny Green fighting pose.

some, and you ate a hamburger and chips and drank some Coke in the chair and afterwards had a nice rest on Dad's lap. Katrina visited, as well as Carolyn, James and Charlotte. Mitchell was not well, so he missed their visit, as he was asleep in the unit. I'll take him home tomorrow and Dad will spend some more time with him, as Grandma is away.

I feel confident we are starting on a new three-month phase in your care and we are looking forward to the rehab element in this. I have brought a lot of toys in so that we can be busy in the mornings with games. You have a wonderful selection of books, DVDs and videos. Along with the play therapist, I think we will get by. I'll arrange the music therapist too. We plan to do a dressing change every four days; this will give you enough of a break so that you are not fasted and you get the necessary feeds. You are strong-minded and loud – we see this as a sign that you are getting better.

Carolyn's journal, Day 86, Saturday 13 March 2004
Sophie lay in my lap this morning and Mitchell and Ron, Sophie and I watched videos; it was nice. Ron has agreed to spend a couple of nights at home next week as part of the new plan to spend more time at home for Mitchell and his work. Peter has suggested another graft next Wednesday and hopefully having Sophie fully grafted in four weeks. I feel we are progressing towards a healthy routine for Sophie, giving her more time to rest and maintain her feeds.

Ron's journal, Day 86, Saturday 13 March 2004
Woke up with Mitchell and he had a temperature of thirty-nine. I gave him paracetamol and it went down pretty quickly. Went and had breakfast with Mitchell and then went to see Sophie. Caro seemed fairly relaxed.

Letter to Sophie, Day 87, Sunday 14 March 2004
I'm sleeping with you tonight after a good day. You sat in your chair and did some hand exercises, and you did good rolling in your bed when you had another rectal tube in, so you got to choose a sticker to put on your Barbie calendar. You slept from 7.30 until 8.30. Now, it's just after ten and you are so itchy, you are very agitated. Rod Smith and his daughter Mikala visited today; she drew some beautiful pictures for you. She brought stories in to read but you had just done a big poo so it wasn't the best time. I see the need for you to re-learn every small movement, as if you were a six-month-old learning to grasp objects. You get frustrated at what you can't do, and say, 'I'm sad.' We have to persevere, so I have brought in an additional range of activities to give us some variety. Mitchell was very excited because Dad was going to sleep at home – the first time since the accident. He keeps planning activities we can do when you get out of hospital. He misses you terribly and misses our family life, as we all do. We will have it again soon for your sake and his. xo

Carolyn's journal, Day 87, Sunday 14 March 2004
A sad day. I cried in the car after dropping Mitchell home. So many reminders of how happy our life was. Mitch and I went to Trudy's baby shower – shades of three years ago, when we expected three weeks between our babies' arrivals and we ended up with Zach and Sophie on the same day! I was listening to Linda and Carolyn plan Easter holidays and knowing that for us, this year will be one of hospital life. I mourn the loss of our beautiful family. These are the days when loneliness and sorrow descend and are all-pervasive. I yearn for joy to enter my heart again.

Letter to Sophie, Day 88, Monday 15 March 2004
Mary came to visit, which was good since she could lend a

hand. Dad arrived to you coming back from a dressing change agitated and unsettled, which took six and a half hours to work through. Before this, your day was a good one; you sat on my lap and we watched videos. You drew your first picture and it was wonderful. We gave it to Dr Andy, whose birthday is on 9 April; he kept reminding you that you both had birthdays coming up. You saw a McDonald's ad on TV and wanted McDonald's for lunch, then just before you went to sleep again you asked for McDonald's – the power of advertising. Dad almost forgot the toy, though; he was in big trouble from me and had to go and rectify it because you asked him for 'my toy' in the dressing change. Your hand is healing well and we will wait till Thursday to find out how your leg went. Although Daddy said he didn't sleep that well last night, I know it gave him great pleasure being at home. I hope that we can do some appropriate renovations to this house so that we can return to a stable environment and settle into our new life sometime in the future. My brave princess.

Carolyn's journal, Day 88, Monday 15 March 2004
A lovely day – till 3 pm, when Sophie returned completely unsettled from a dressing change. Again, we gave as much medicine as we could, but Sophie could not settle, and it is so distressing seeing her go through this and not knowing what else can be done.

I met Sandra in the kitchen today and gave her my thoughts on our new family timetable, my pain at our loss and how I am looking forward to our future in our new home. I feel I can see a dim light at the end of the tunnel. Peter Hayward spoke to me about the pace slowing for grafting; it's a matter of priorities in theatre and, as Peter says, Sophie is a survivor and there are more life-threatening operations that have to take priority. I understand that because we have been there.

Letter to Sophie, Day 89, Tuesday 16 March 2004
Today, Louise stayed reading stories with you while Daddy and I attended doctors' meetings. We had a follow-up meeting with the pain team. They tried to assess why you were so unsettled after your dressing change yesterday. You wanted Linda to visit and I saw lovely spontaneous play and smiles, with a tea party and lots of cooking. You got quite sad when she left and wanted her back 'now!'. You have a plaster cast on your hand so that you can extend your fingers to ninety degrees; it's really important to your grip. I stroke your tummy as I convince you to close your eyes, because it's 10.45 and you need to be asleep. At last, you rest easy – the light is low and your lullaby CD is on. You wake with a start from time to time and I just reassure you that things are okay. A small morphine bolus means that you sleep without noticing the pain in your ear, shoulder and tummy. It's so nice to see you rested and comfortable, and I figured out how to fix your bed so it had the ripple mode, allowing you a massage effect and release from pressure-point areas. Here's hoping for a settled night – in some fashion. I smother you in rainbows!

Carolyn's journal, Day 89, Tuesday 16 March 2004
Today, only eleven different doctors/teams visited but up to three nurses at once, at least every fifteen to thirty minutes throughout the day. They are all keeping a discreet distance from Sophie so she is not overloaded (my theory is that she has sensory overload).

Letter to Sophie, Day 90, Wednesday 17 March 2004
Today, we took your rectal tube out. A lot of time is wasted with the flush that could be better used with physio, etc. We got you into your chair; your tummy is a bit unsettled and you vomit a lot of the meds, but there are a lot needed. It's a vicious cycle and

I have no immediate answer. It will just be that the better you get, the less you will need. Your plaster cast is assisting a range of movements with your left hand. Dr Andy was thrilled with the drawing we gave him of Dorothy the Dinosaur. You sleep listening to a CD on rainbows. We are collecting a lot of rainbow cards as well as your ribbons and the wonderful rainbow that Mitchell painted. I love the calm in your room tonight; here's hoping it continues to the wee small hours. You have had one antibiotic withdrawn. We like that; we're praying it won't be needed again. You are an inspiration and so wonderfully courageous. I can't tell you how proud of you I am.

Ron's journal, Day 90, Wednesday 17 March 2004
Woke up in the middle of the night not knowing where I was. It seemed so surreal that over at the hospital there was Sophie and Caro, and I was in my own bed in my own home.

Letter to Sophie, Day 91, Thursday 18 March 2004
A wonderful day. You went outside. You received a balloon and a small radio because they launched the marketing for the Easter Show at the hospital. You played lots of games with Lisa and did beautiful paintings. We have four of them on the wall in lovely silver frames. You were happy and interactive, which was wonderful to see. We had cables running everywhere outside the door with all your monitors; you wanted to go for a slide, which we said you could do soon.

We have been waiting for your theatre time for grafts to your shoulder and right elbow – scheduled for 9 am, so you have been fasted since 2 am. You end up going to theatre at 3.30 pm. You are agitated post-op and we try everything to get you to sleep. Kam Soon came to see you at 11 pm and gave you a big hit of morphine to get you off to sleep. Last night, you slept from 7.30

pm to 8.30 am with only four wakes – your best sleep in three and a half months of hospital stay – and while we couldn't hope for a similar night, I hope you stay rested, because you will be a much happier girl.

Carolyn's journal, Day 91, Thursday 18 March 2004
Yet another day of fasting, when feeds are critical. A wonderful sleep meant Sophie was in a good mood all day, except for wanting water. We wheeled her bed outside, and Lisa the play therapist did painting. Post-surgery another traumatic time, with Sophie unsettled, crying and agitated. David Murrell stayed with her in recovery because he had administered more anaesthetic than he had ever given to a child and was concerned.

Ron's journal, Day 91, Thursday 18 March 2004
Operation day today. Sophie is going in for dressing change and a skin graft to cover her shoulders and a few other spots on her legs and elbow. Sophie was in such good spirits in the morning. I was at home last night to spend a bit of time with Mitchell before going back to the hospital in the afternoon. Got the call from Caro saying that it was going to be a 9 am operation instead of an afternoon operation. I quickly got showered and dressed and rushed back to the hospital.

The traffic was horrendous and I arrived back at 9.30 am, to find that Sophie still hadn't gone into theatre. The operation ended up happening at 3.30 pm. Spoke to Andy, who said that the previous skin grafts went very well, with all the grafts taking. Caro left the hospital around 12.30 pm to go to work and then to collect Mitchell. I spoke to her in the afternoon and we decided that she would spend the night with Mitchell at home. I'm sure they needed the time at home together. It made me feel better, as I was a bit guilty about spending three nights at home during the week.

Caro finishes one journal and starts another; this seems to coincide with a turning point in Sophie's recovery.

Letter to Sophie, Day 92, Friday 19 March 2004
We turn the corner and turn the book! This morning, you did a big catch-up sleep-in till lunchtime. You had a happy afternoon, waking up after all that sleep in a good mood. Mitchell and I headed home, as I had some work to do invoicing, but all I did was tidy your bedroom. You have bags of soft toys everywhere, some lovely dolls and games to come home to. Your bed is filled with bears. I want to get Dad to photograph it so we can show you. I tidied Mitchell's room, too, and Daddy and I decided it would be okay for me to stay the night at home – my first time for three and a half months.

Mitchell and I had a bath, then we had dinner with Grandpa and our usual routine of stories and bed for Mitchell. It was good to be home but I'd almost forgotten which cupboard the plates were kept in! It was 1 am before I got to sleep because it was so quiet: there were no monitors beeping, no nurses in and out of the room and a comfortable bed – all quite different. All around, there were reminders of you but I know that we will be taking you home soon and it will be joyous.

Carolyn's journal, Day 92, Friday 19 March 2004
A sleepy morning post-surgery, which is usual for Sophie. Ron stayed with Sophie as I took Mitchell home – we tidied his room and then I started on Sophie's. It was great therapy. We had a ball together and the usual bedtime routine. Even so, it felt as though there was an almighty gap in everything I did.

Ron's journal, Day 92, Friday 19 March 2004
The night was okay. Sophie woke a couple of times for a nappy change and around eight times either thirsty or because of the nurses: some nurses just walk in the room and are noisy, while others take care. The day went well, with Russell coming over

for a cup of coffee. A couple of weeks back, Russell brought his son Aaron over. Aaron had sixty-five per cent burns twenty years ago. Russell said that after their visit to us, Aaron seemed to face his demons and realised what Russell had to go through when he was just two. Russell thanked me and said that Aaron wanted now to do something for other kids with burns. I took Russell over to meet Sandra for a chat. I hope Aaron gets involved, as he seems a great kid.

Caro and Mitch came over in the afternoon, with Mitchell in good spirits. I also spoke to Melissa Cooke [friend] about getting the Wiggles over to see Sophie for her birthday. She said she would chase them up but found out later that they are in the USA and England over April. I need to do something special for Sophie for this, her third birthday.

Letter to Sophie, Day 93, Saturday 20 March 2004

I cried all the way back to the hospital today. I cried for you and for our happy life lost. I cried because I was afraid of the future, for you having to go through more hurt. If anyone can do it, you can, because ever since you were a baby your strong personality has shone through. Ever since you could talk, you were decisive in everything you did. You taught me a lot and continue to do so. You surprise and delight me with everything you do at the moment. Today, when John and Kate visited and blew bubbles, one landed in your eye. I washed it with water. Earlier, I had shown you your sunglasses, among other things I had brought from home for you. You said, 'I want wear my sunglasses,' so that the bubbles didn't go in your eyes. It made everyone laugh.

We had a pizza PJ party tonight, with Beth in your room. Your grafts on your shoulders have limited the amount of movement we can do, so we have activities in your bed instead. Your arm is in plaster, so we cannot do much with your fingers, and you get frustrated when you can't complete a task or game. We don't want you getting upset, so we quickly switch games to something you enjoy, or find another way of playing it so that it is not as frustrating. Your independence shines through as always.

Carolyn's journal, Day 93, Saturday 20 March 2004
I swam in the morning and completed some invoicing – felt like I had achieved something but cried all the way back to hospital. Sophie had lots of visitors and I sense she was quite tired at the end of it all. She stayed awake till 10.30 pm and had a disturbed sleep, not particularly deep. Her tummy is sore and she was agitated.

Ron's journal, Day 93, Saturday 20 March 2004
Mitchell is going to the zoo today with Melissa and the other parents from the Roundhouse. Sophie was pretty good last night – not too many wake-ups but enough to make it a broken sleep. I still find it amazing how Sophie takes it. She has been in pain on and off for ninety-seven days, with the occasional smile and laugh! Allan brought Mitchell back around 3.30 pm; Allan was exhausted.

Letter to Sophie, Day 94, Sunday 21 March 2004
You had a quiet morning and a sleepy afternoon. Grandma Joy arrived back from New Zealand and it was wonderful to see her. Mitchell was very excited. Catherine came to see you and you slept through the whole visit. It is proving difficult to draw blood from your central line, which is a problem that will continue to resurface. Dr Andy has spoken of the next graft and the need to position you prone for two weeks. We will have to have significant consultation on how we best manage

that process. Mitchell misses you very much and it's sad. We walked along the corridor the other day and he said, pointing to the space between him and me, 'The only thing that is missing just there is Sophie.' He gave you a drink today and was very gentle in how he tended to you. Your good-natured spirit inspires everyone, and people are pleased to be around you and working with you to help you get well. Daddy said when we get home you can go shopping to buy anything you like. You said chocolate and clothes.

Carolyn's journal, Day 94, Sunday 21 March 2004
Nurse Susan was on. She's lovely – concerned about Sophie's back and oozing. Dressing done and Sophie went prone – this was all after a big nappy change. Sophie is grumpy – still tired, sore tummy, looking pale. Could be an upset tummy. We cannot rule out anything as a possibility. Temp at 38.7 degrees yesterday, up to thirty-nine! I hope her line is not causing problems again. She was in a happier mood when she woke this time and the humour is shining through.

Letter to Sophie, Day 95, Monday 22 March 2004
This morning, you had a dressing change. Daddy juggled balls. I read you your Tigger story from Auntie Ann-Louise, and Lisa showed you all sorts of coloured toys that had liquid in them and moved about – magic wands, water wheels, etc. It took one and a half hours for your legs, head and back to be re-dressed. You managed exceptionally well, I think. Lyn read you stories after lunch. Dr Andy came to draw blood from your problem central line. The doctor from the pain team reported in on pain management and we put you prone. You will go prone for a few hours every day again so that your back can heal. The cultured skin cells are more delicate and it will just be a longer process.

I think we have three grafts left and it will take six weeks at best. Michelle [physiotherapist] wants to have you in the chair and more mobile again tomorrow after last week's graft to your shoulders. Your patience is undeniable, your spirit determined. You have lost none of your decisiveness, and your trust in those around you helping you is ever present. You are my brave, courageous girl.

Carolyn's journal, Day 95, Monday 22 March 2004
Sophie is adamant that she wants to hold the thermometer in her hand herself. Temp is up to 39.3 degrees. I've noticed the temps creeping up, so I hope it's not another infection. Sophie is amazing how she copes with being prone, her personality shining through despite the most obvious difficulties. Sophie asked about her nasal prongs yesterday – 'What are they? Why?' – an indication that she is more aware. She asked tonight where Daddy was sleeping. I said, 'In the hospital bedroom.' She said, 'Where is it?' I said, 'Along the corridor.'

Dreadful noises from other crying children distress everyone – nurses included.

Ron's journal, Day 95, Monday 22 March 2004
Had [nurse X] last night. She had to replace the morphine and had trouble getting it to work. I could see the problem myself. Sophie was in a lot of pain for around an hour. We found blood on the sheets where the line connections were and blood in the line to the body side. I told the nurse that obviously the morphine's not going in. She argued with me and then tightened up all the connections, and the blood went from the lines. Other than that, Sophie slept fairly well. I say this keeping in mind I had to wake around thirty-five times during the night for all the nappy changes or Sophie needing either pain relief or just assurance that all is okay. Left for home to be with Mitchell. Caro to do the night shift.

chapter nine
one hundred days

In this marathon strewn with miracles, the Delezio family reach the hundred-day mark. Carolyn and Ron seem to find a new surge of strength as they start to see 'more upsides than downsides' in Sophie's recovery.

Letter to Sophie, Day 96, Tuesday 23 March 2004
You have your sight, your hearing, your sense of smell, the ability to taste, to speak and sing. God chose you on 15 December to live. Your determination shines through everything you do. Today, we tried to take blood from your central line, so we had you doing all sorts of exercises to your Hooley Dooleys video. Your arms were marching in front of you at ninety degrees. We laid you prone to take blood and I asked you to move your shoulders back and forth, and you did. You try so hard. You did beautiful finger-paintings and used the play dough with Lisa today to make sausages and balls. You cut play

vegetables with a knife. We sent one of your paintings off with Andy to Concord Hospital. Viv [friend] came to sit with you while you slept and then played again with you and Michelle during physio. Dr Andy and Dr Hayward came to visit and you went all quiet. Beckie and Tricia came to visit from PICU today – you cried when Tricia left. She is special to you.

Carolyn's journal, Day 96, Tuesday 23 March 2004
Pain team reviewed today, as did the gastro team; a scan has been ordered. We are completing an abdominal chart to track tummy pain. Sophie's central line didn't bleed, despite moving positions, arm exercises and going prone. A doctor had to come and take blood via a finger prick. Soph will have a test for her line on Wednesday to see if we can salvage it prior to Thursday. If not, a femoral line will be required.

Ron's journal, Day 96, Tuesday 23 March 2004
Couldn't sleep last night. Had Mitchell in bed with me, and he sleeps all over the place. I'm one of these people who can't stand anything touching me while I sleep. Not only that, it is getting used to a different bed, a different pillow – and the quiet.

Got dressed and took Mitchell to school. He was very quiet when we got there. I know that after a while he'll be okay. Went back home and did some work. Also went to the real-estate agent, just in case we need to move house. Linda and Wayne came over for a barbecue. Had a good night, finished off with a nice hot spa with Allan till around 11.30 pm. What a different world we were in compared with the hospital. So surreal. I just couldn't believe what had happened, really happened. During the day, we had our staff meeting with the physio, nurses, therapy, etc. Complained about [nurse X] and felt better.

Letter to Sophie, Day 97, Wednesday 24 March 2004
Today, we started with visits from Andy, the pain team, Infectious Diseases, dietician, physio, play therapist, doctor and commenced finger-painting again after Michelle took off your plaster – we are having a break from it tonight. Carolyn came over and stayed with you and Lisa; Nadia, the occupational therapist, also came to observe. You are lying prone tonight to help your back. Your tummy ache has lessened but you vomited quite a bit. You also had a linogram [a scan to see your central line] and a scan of your gall bladder, kidneys and liver. You were so good throughout both.

You sat in your chair today and watched videos with Lyn while I had a massage (so did Grandma). Tonight, Catherine and [her son] Antoni visited, and Maree; you had a little sleep, then watched a DVD with Maree while I had dinner. You are heading to theatre tomorrow with the possibility of a new line going in and a dressing change. I will be going home to be with Mitchell, and he will come out on Friday with me. I hope you have a restful sleep tonight. You deserve it, as it has been a busy day yet again.

With love and admiration, Mummy. x

Carolyn's journal, Day 97, Wednesday 24 March 2004
Finger-painting with Lisa was great today; Soph really loves to paint. Carolyn was over and more games played. OT and physio were happy with progress on fingers and hand, though wrist still tight. Scan for bladder, kidney and liver showed nothing too peculiar – bumpy bits around liver and enlarged kidney due to meds, most likely. The day seems to tumble by without a break. Always so much to achieve in the day but small progressive steps are being made.

Ron's journal, Day 97, Wednesday 24 March 2004
Slept well last night – this time with Mitchell in his own bed. Did some work till around 12 noon and went back to the hospital

as Sophie had some tests. We then had a meeting with Andy and Peter re the central line. We agreed that we will need to put in a new line tomorrow during theatre. Sophie otherwise had a good day, with plenty of smiles and a bit of laughter. Organised a meeting with *60 Minutes* for this afternoon; it was a good meeting with Liz Hayes, Cliff, Lincoln and the hospital.

Letter to Sophie, Day 98, Thursday 25 March 2004
Today was a sleepy day. You didn't feel much like finger-painting but sat on my knee and we had a nice rest/sleep together till Dad arrived. You had been fasted since 2 am, as you are awaiting surgery – a new dressing change and central line, which will be femoral; it's antiseptic coated.

You go to theatre at 4.30 pm. You are grafted again and thrash around a bit with the Medaz given. It made me think that for your next operation we will need a good pain-management strategy pre-op and post-op. You settle finally at 9 pm and wake every half-hour during the night – it was Dad's turn. I was due to go home to spend time with Mitchell, who by the time I arrived had already gone to bed. We are designing a special headrest for you to go prone and checking on equipment that may allow you a degree of flexibility, with a range of movement, when you are prone.

Ron's journal, Day 98, Thursday 25 March 2004
Last night was a better night but had to get going as Sophie was in theatre today. I let Caro go in with Sophie this time, as Sophie wanted her mum. Caro came out and we went back to the unit and made love. Seems a bit strange with Sophie being in theatre but the whole thing is so strange and different that there is no standard thing to do. We hardly ever get a chance to be together these days.

one hundred days

Sophie came out very disturbed afterwards. This time, it was due to the Medazolan after theatre. It took a good couple of hours for her to settle down. Dropped into the golf club and ordered the golf buggy and picked up the golf shirt signed by Annika Sörenstam, Karrie Webb and Laura Davies. This will be auctioned at a charity dinner Friday week.

Letter to Sophie, Day 99, Friday 26 March 2004
I was thrilled to see you so happy this afternoon/evening. I think it's the happiest and best spirited I have seen you in hospital. You surprise everyone with your good spirits.

Mitchell and I spent a lovely morning swimming in the pool, playing on the swings and wishing you were with us. We went swimming with Grandma Joy. I took photos of your room today so Dad could print them out and put them on your wall. You received a lovely parcel from the Roundhouse, with more toys, puzzles and games. This will help keep you entertained for the next few months. You cried when Granny Lyn left; you slept well with her this afternoon while Dad and I had meetings. A new splint is being made for your legs to keep them in position – i.e. not bent; this will give the best result for your prosthetic limbs. We had a happy time in your room this evening – all having dinner, then reading stories and watching videos. You were so happy.

Lisa dropped around a photo of you today balancing a ball on your head – it's priceless. She'd balanced the ball on her head first, apparently, and you'd laughed so much at her when she was doing it that you'd wanted to do it too.

Your room is looking like an art gallery with all your finger-painting masterpieces. You are getting requests from all around the hospital for your artwork, so we'll be very busy next week. When you're happy, we are all happy. It's a joy to see. Love you. x

Carolyn's journal, Day 99, Friday 26 March 2004
Mitchell and I stay and play in the house. I don't get much done around the place but have a lovely time relaxing with Mitch, Mum and Dad. Sophie is in a really happy mood this afternoon/evening. We have meetings with Carrie and physio. We had dinner in Sophie's room and Mitchell played with toys and drew. He was the best he has been in her room.

Ron's journal, Day 99, Friday 26 March 2004
I felt like a zombie this morning. Spoke to Caro and told her to take it easy and spend some time at home. Had a good morning with Sophie. Lyn took care of Sophie for a couple of hours and I went back to the room for a break. Caro can definitely handle sleep deprivation better than I can. Found out today that Mum has been pretty bad with her arthritis and Dad had collapsed on the floor [he had fainted after a long bout of coughing had hampered his breathing]. Normally, I would have been around straight away but times are now different. I spoke to Mum and Dad on the phone anyway. Mitchell was very excited about being back at the hospital.

Letter to Sophie, Day 100, Saturday 27 March 2004
You had a sleep today, so we left you just to relax and watch videos and DVDs. John and Kate came out to visit, and Linda spent time reading you stories, which you loved. You have vomited quite a bit overnight and today, so we have had to give you anti-nausea medication and something for your itch. When Linda was reading you stories, we spent time with Mitchell and went for a walk with him around the hospital and to Ronald McDonald House for a play. This is a rare time, when we can both be with him. The weather is more comfortable now, so it's nice to go for a walk away from the air conditioning and to feel the breeze. We look

forward to being able to take you for a walk in your wheelchair when you are more mobile. Daddy is sleeping with you tonight, so I left with Mitchell at 8.30 pm to read him stories and tuck him in. He spent all morning in your room doing drawing. He loves doing drawings for you and writing you letters.

Carolyn's journal, Day 100, Saturday 27 March 2004
Diazepam and clonidine and any oral meds are making Sophie vomit, so we ask for ondansetron and Vallergan (meds for anti-nausea and itch). She seems to settle following her broken sleep, waking each hour last night. We have put feeds down to forty [millilitres per hour] and hope she absorbs these better. The adult rate is eighty, so sixty-five is just too high.

Ron's journal, Day 100, Saturday 27 March 2004
What a memorable day – a hundred days of this pain and suffering for Sophie and all of us.

Letter to Sophie, Day 101, Sunday 28 March 2004
Another sleepy day today. You went prone between 9 pm and 2 am, a good stretch, but then said, 'I stuck – I want get off!' when you had had enough. Trudy came with Zach and brought videos and stories. She read to you throughout the afternoon; the baby is due in three weeks. You watched *Peter Rabbit* again and again with her. Grandma and Grandpa came to have a pizza party in your room tonight. Mitchell gets sad when it's time to leave to go back to Baranbali Avenue. Your tummy is sore: sometimes needing to vomit, sometimes itchy, sometimes just sore. Sometimes it's mid-tum, sometimes it's abdo pain. So we give you the appropriate meds and massage with the little hand massager that you like. After waking every hour during the night till 2 am, I try to sleep in the back room of the ward. I can't, so at three I return and you

are having stories read. We settle again at four and you wake with tummy pain at 6.15, sleep again at 6.45 and then sleep through to 10 am. Having your feeds running at forty seems to have slowed the violence of the vomiting. You still vomit after meds, unfortunately, and go 'yuck, yuck, yuck – I don't like it'.

Carolyn's journal, Day 101, Sunday 28 March 2004
Small amounts of physio are done over the weekend. Today, a dressing change with Exu-Dry jacket because of smell and vomit – unscheduled but easy to do while you are prone. It still takes over an hour, though. Bactigrass is put on as the scarlet-red dressing is removed [scarlet red is an ointment used to help the healing process]. Tummy pain wakes Sophie at night. I wake at hourly intervals, then try to sleep in the back room. Ron came in at 6.45, so I went to the room to try to catch a couple more hours. Broken because of constant phone calls.

Letter to Sophie, Day 102, Monday 29 March 2004
You slept till 10 am, when you had Nana and Nanu visit with Auntie Michelle; you were happy and chatty. Lyn was here to sit with you for quiet time and you had a small sleep while I had lunch with Grandma and Grandpa, because Grandpa is going back to New Zealand for two months. You were woken by a doctor who needs to do a finger prick because we can't bleed back off your line.

Catherine and Antoni came by with beautiful big Nemo and Marlin balloons and flowers. So did Trish, who is leaving PICU and Westmead today. She shares your birthday on 3 April and will be thirty-three. She is off to do volunteer work in Africa; I have asked her to keep in touch. You had a urine sample taken for testing. We have fashioned a new pillow for your head, so will see how that goes overnight. Will try to get your feeds up to fifty-six to help you put on weight and get stronger. You throw up after your meds. You want to visit Lilly Fay's house [friend].

Carolyn's journal, Day 102, Monday 29 March 2004
A dressing change at 11 am–12.30 pm, with morphine bolus and nitrous oxide. Sophie managed really well. Lisa blows bubbles and distracts and is a great support. Orthotics came down to measure splints, which have been made and will need to be worn in anticipation of prosthetic limbs being made.

Letter to Sophie, Day 103, Tuesday 30 March 2004
A lovely, restful sleep overnight and we lay together and watched cartoons in the morning. Your plaster cast came off and we got you into your chair for playtime with Lisa – cooking, finger-paint and dough. You had a very happy time. We will push your birthday party out one week. An Exu-Dry jacket and dressing change front and back agitated you after a lovely story/chat time with Mary. It took about six hours to settle you into a disturbed sleep.

We had you prone for three and a half hours and will need to work on getting your splint in place overnight again. Your feeds are running at fifty and you seem to tolerate this well. Peter Hayward called by and he is very happy with your tummy, so the graft will go ahead when PICU have a bed available. Your range of movements is improving and when I sat outside for a meeting today you waved your purple hand at me because you don't want to wash your finger-paint off your fingers.

Carolyn's journal, Day 103, Tuesday 30 March 2004
Usual Tuesday meeting occurred, with some progress towards a coordinated plan for Sophie's next graft and housekeeping matters. Had a meeting with orthotics and OT re limb deficiency,

particulars with the house and speed with which she will learn to walk, how often to expect to wear legs (inside), going outside in a wheelchair, and maybe later a scooter.

Letter to Sophie, Day 104, Wednesday 31 March 2004
We had the *60 Minutes* crew here while you were watching *Playschool*. They left us in peace while we did a nappy change, then came to film you playing with Lisa – you were lifted into your chair. Nadia from OT brought a special yellow table for you. You did finger-painting, cooking and playing with goop. We gave you a bowl of water and cotton-wool balls to wash your hand with. Your right hand was covered in a glove and you enjoyed painting with it. You played with plastic fish floating in water. You sat in your chair for five and a half hours with a couple of sleeps and at the end your bottom was sore. So it was back to bed, after a cuddle with me while your bed was made.

We had your oxygen-mask nasal prongs off for half an hour and your rate was eighty-eight. Catherine and Lee visited, as did Damian, your doctor who worked with Peter Hayward in the first month. He came with Andy and was clearly emotional when he left. I gave him a 'Journey' T-shirt because he played a vital role. We had a lovely night up until our bedtime. We played push-button games and I did a little tidying up. We had the 'going on a bear hunt' story three times and hid under the blankets in our 'cubby'. We watched the stars on your ceiling and you sang songs as I lay next to you in your bed. It was a very special, magical night, which I will treasure always.

Carolyn's journal, Day 104, Wednesday 31 March 2004
Nadia has a special table for Sophie with a cut-out tummy; it allows her elbows to rest on it, so it can be raised to allow a range of movement of ninety degrees. Sophie used her right arm

well and in the evening was even more comfortable, moving her arms around. Sophie is allowed two to three hours out of a cast on her left arm during playtime.

Letter to Sophie, Day 105, Thursday 1 April 2004
An early start, with *60 Minutes* filming our morning wake-up, physio session and play session, all in anticipation of another theatre trip. Today, you went to theatre for a dressing change, new central line, catheter, NG tube and ultrasound on your heart. Unfortunately, your new central line didn't transpire, because of blocked veins; we will have to troubleshoot our way out of this situation. You played so nicely today with Lisa, despite being tired, and did beautiful bubble-blowing with your sunglasses and hat on.

David Murrell had a new strategy after theatre, with a dose of ketamine running through your morphine. This seems to be working well and it is the most settled we have seen you post-op for some weeks. Louise visited today with a range of musical wind instruments that I'm looking forward to using with you. Mitchell stayed with Grandma Joy because of theatre, so he will only have two days at hospital this week. Dad and I played in your cubby house this morning and you had the best smile on your face when I pretended I couldn't find you or Daddy. You are moving both your arms about very well, more than you ever had before, and it's wonderful to see you gaining confidence. Maybe we can go outside tomorrow.

Carolyn's journal, Day 105, Thursday 1 April 2004
Sophie's arm movements and bubble-blowing today are the best we've seen. It's hard to know what to plan for Sophie's birthday because we don't know when she will be called to have another graft – it's dependent on PICU beds. There is a lot of politics at

play at the moment, with PICU being full of children who are not going anywhere in a hurry.

Letter to Sophie, Day 106, Friday 2 April 2004
After a few vomits this morning, we settled into a morning of physio; the splint came off and exercises were done. I suggested getting into bed behind you to have you sitting more upright. So I hopped into bed and we had a lovely couple of hours. You were very tired from theatre the previous day, so you didn't interact with Lisa much but had a relaxed sleep. You were more upright than you would have been in your chair. Our aim is to have you support your head more, maybe with a neck roll.

Lyn came, and Mitchell and I went shopping for birthday presents, wrapping paper and cards. We had dinner in your room, watched movies and Mitchell coloured in. It was lovely to be able to do that as a family. You ate some chicken, which was good, and fell quietly asleep. We left Dad to turn you prone when it was appropriate, having put your creams on and chosen your special oil for your wheat pillow [a small cushion that can be used as a hot pack or a cold pack]. Catherine came to visit after the charity lunch held at Star City, with funds going to the trust. The public support is simply amazing.

Carolyn's journal, Day 106, Friday 2 April 2004
A rested night. Prone for ten and a half hours, which is a fantastic result – the ketamine and morphine worked well. Lyn was in to sit with Sophie over lunch, while Mitchell and I went shopping for Sophie's birthday. Mitchell drew on the leather lounge at home today – a cry for attention. We had dinner in Sophie's room, watching movies. She was asleep but Mitchell told me he went up and held her hand. Overall, more upsides than downsides this week.

one hundred days

chapter ten
Sophie is three

'A third birthday that we thought we would not see with our little girl,' writes Carolyn. Even in a hospital room, surrounded by all the smells, sights and sounds of the medical world that is now hers, Sophie is as excited as any birthday girl could be. She is surrounded by presents, a party atmosphere and people who love her.

The ongoing cycle of grafts means that Sophie must return to PICU for a time. Once she is back in the Burns ward, though, she shows her energy and determination by kicking her legs. After many months of immobility, she clearly wants to be on the move.

Ron stops keeping a journal around this time. In one of his last entries, he notes the difference that antidepressants have made to him in gaining a new perspective on Sophie's accident and her injuries: counting their blessings, rather than dwelling on what they have lost.

Letter to Sophie, Day 107, Saturday 3 April 2004
Your third birthday. What a wonderfully happy day this was.

The nurses made you a special card and you were given a toy cash register – something you have always wanted. Mitchell and I arrived, and we opened presents; he helped you and you ripped some paper too. He was very excited, as were you – your eyes were bright and cheerful. You did your exercises, you had a change of dressing on your head and then you were all set to wear your beautiful fairy dress that Joan had made for you. Joan is one of the wonderful volunteers in the shop upstairs, who went out of her way to make something that would work for you to wear.

Catherine, Antoni and his friend Blake were at your party – so were Grandma Joy, Linda, Wayne and Lillie [friend], Mandy and Margaret Henry, Lee and Mark, Melissa, Michael, Justin and Jessica Cooke [friends], Maree, Scott and Lilly and Caroline and Molly. Maree was the fairy godmother 'Magic Maree' and Louise brought all the balloons; Captain Starlight came and did magic tricks for you too. We had pass the parcel and Melissa had arranged party bags. Dot had made you a beautiful Dorothy the Dinosaur birthday cake and it was the only time you cried – characteristic of a three-year-old. You were chatty and happy throughout the day, though. You ate Cheezels and chips and drank Coke – typical party treats. *60 Minutes* filmed. John and Kate, William and Oliver were with you as well for the afternoon. You truly shone like a star.

Carolyn's journal, Day 107, Saturday 3 April 2004
And a third birthday that we thought we would not see with our little girl. We wanted the girls to share a small party, so Caroline and Scott, Molly and Lilly came to visit in the afternoon. This all followed a good physio session and a head-dressing change. Happy, chatty and enjoying the party – that's how I would sum up Sophie's day.

Ron's journal, Day 107, Saturday 3 April 2004
Sophie's birthday today. She's so excited. It's so good to see our

little girl still getting excited, even though under her bandages she is so extremely hurt. Sophie ended up with three cakes: one Dorothy cake, one ice-cream cake and another from Trudy (on Sunday). We filled her room with helium balloons and we all played pass the parcel around Sophie's bed, Sophie included.

Letter to Sophie, Day 108, Sunday 4 April 2004
Ron said you had an unsettled night – probably too many chips and Cheezels at your party. Katrina and John, Trudy and Zach came to visit, and Katrina said you had a happy day. I spent it at home taking Mitchell to a party and hooking up for a chat with the US branch of the family.

A few domestic duties and a trip to the museum with Grandma filled the day. Mitchell and I did a few puzzles, and it was sad leaving him at home. Grandma told me Auntie Ann-Louise has booked a house at Collaroy in July for three weeks. That will be fantastic: it's on the beachfront, so there will be wonderful walks and lots of rock pools to explore. Grandpa Allan has gone back to New Zealand for two months; Uncle Greg said he spoke to him and he is enjoying being back home with a cocktail in hand watching the tide coming in and the sun setting. We will have to arrange a special thank you for your birthday for Mum; she has put in a big effort in looking after us all. You look beautiful and we are about to put you prone for the evening.

Carolyn's journal, Day 108, Sunday 4 April 2004
After putting Mitchell to bed with two stories, I sat with Mum and we had a chat and a cuppa – probably the first time we've done this one-on-one since the accident. Up early for a computer hook-up with the US. It was good to see them all again. Mitchell off to party; I went home and met Rebecca [Riddington]. I became teary when Rebecca recounted the public support for the girls.

I did a few domestic chores while Mitchell was at the party. Then, Mum and I picked him up and we went to the museum, then back home before I left for the hospital. It was awful leaving Mitchell – he was sad but brave and I felt sorrow for our fragmented family. I cried on the way back to hospital again. Sophie was a little sad for the first hour of my return, so I opened some more birthday presents with her and she cheered up. She loves to watch the Olympic swimming trials on TV.

Letter to Sophie, Day 109, Monday 5 April 2004
After a reasonable night, we got ready for a full dressing change, and it was in the bath – your first bath with bubbles and a rubber duck, in what's called the shower bath. This took two hours, then we sat with you in your room till you slept. All was well until meds went in and the magnesium made you vomit. You brought up the Vegemite sandwich you had for lunch. Later, we had a little cuddle, with me sitting behind you this evening. It's lovely having that time with you, helping you get more upright and more used to being handled.

Carolyn's journal, Day 109, Monday 5 April 2004
I'm tired and sad and feel the effects of only having half an hour out of the room today. Sophie's first bath went well, although it was a long dressing change. We still await a theatre time for her graft this week.

Letter to Sophie, Day 110, Tuesday 6 April 2004
A broken night's sleep left us both pretty tired, but you sat in your chair for about five hours. I tried to do some tidying up in the unit today because I had just dumped bags after

Saturday's party. I got back to the room for 3 pm, when Ron had arranged a meeting with Jenny Ault (the rehab specialist) and the occupational therapist. I sat behind you again to get you more upright and you kept asking to watch the swimming, but the Olympic trials have finished and you are very disappointed.

We are still unwrapping birthday presents. Beckie from PICU came down to visit and to give you a Noddy DVD, which you love. You are a little sad because you say you miss Daddy and Mitchell. We start getting ready for bed at 8.45 pm and after a nappy change and meds you are ready for 9.30. By the time we settle for the night – I sleep when you do – it's 10 pm. We will have to get earlier nights so we can get up earlier in the mornings! I feel sad for you tonight and sometimes I feel sad for us and that we miss each other so . . . it won't be long, though!

Carolyn's journal, Day 110, Tuesday 6 April 2004
Up at ten, which meant we had a busy morning, with physio, Lisa, pain team, Infectious Diseases, Dr Andy and dietician all visiting before twelve. Lyn came in and I snuck away for a shower before the group meeting. Morphine lowered during the day so it can be doubled at night.

Letter to Sophie, Day 111, Wednesday 7 April 2004
A really good night prone – ten hours but a sleepy morning. Mind you, it was 10 pm when we got to sleep last night. I sat behind you to do things with Lisa, but you were pretty tired and wanted Lisa to do all the work.

Grandma Joy came to visit as well as Lyn; we left you watching your new Noddy DVD from Beckie. Catherine came and apparently you watched it three times while Grandma and I cleaned the apartment and did some washing and tidying up.

Lisa came back to check if you wanted to do anything around three but you weren't really interested as Lyn had brought in a texture bag of goodies, which you played with. Lisa has made a texture 'We're going on a lion hunt' book, which you love running your hands over.

I left to pick up Mitchell and we were having dinner when Daddy rang to say surgery was scheduled for 10 am. It was funny sleeping in our own bed; I woke up at 3 am and had difficulty going back to sleep. I missed you and I missed caring for you, although I knew Daddy was doing a great job.

Carolyn's journal, Day 111, Wednesday 7 April 2004
Woke Sophie with a finger prick to get a cross-match for theatre tomorrow. Back to see Soph for an hour before Ron arrived and I headed home to pick up Mitchell. A call from Ron saying it's not afternoon but morning for surgery tomorrow – means my relaxing morning at home will not eventuate. No hot water for my relaxing bath, either! We are fine-tuning all the requirements for physio post-op and over Easter, with foam neck-brace pieces in place to make you as comfortable as possible. Ron said Kam Soon came to say farewell, as he is off to Concord.

Letter to Sophie, Day 112, Thursday 8 April 2004
Mitchell and I arrived when you were due for theatre but your time was changed to the afternoon. It was great, because Mitchell got time to spend in your room with you. Then you saw Captain Starlight and wanted to talk to him, so Daddy rang him and asked if the Easter Bunny could come and bring you Easter eggs. Soon enough, he was down to visit with an Easter basket and guitar in hand. He sang 'Twinkle Twinkle', 'Old MacDonald', 'Puff the Magic Dragon' and 'In The Jungle'. You sang with him. He blew you a kiss when he was going and you

blew him one back. Then, as soon as Mitchell and Daddy got back to the room, you told them as proud as punch about the Captain's visit. We were called for theatre at 3 pm; you were grafted on your back and head and a new central line put in. We have brought some of your things [to PICU] from your room on Clubbe Ward.

Carolyn's journal, Day 112, Thursday 8 April 2004
Arrived back to hospital to be told surgery is 1 pm. It gave us a great opportunity to read and play. I particularly wanted Mitchell to spend time with Sophie before the operation. It was still tenuous at 2.30 as to whether Soph would be admitted to PICU, as beds were stretched again. We were discussing plan B with Peter Hayward but a call was made and availability of a bed confirmed. It was all go from that point: Mitchell came to theatre, I went into the theatre consulting room and Sophie cried and said, 'I'm scared.' We did visualisations and went to her safe and happy place, which for Sophie is her pool. It breaks your heart – you want to take the pain, fear and anguish away. At 7 pm, the theatre is over and a good surgical result is given by Peter.

It brings back all the intense emotions of previous visits to PICU – especially today, when Brian told us he was taking Ben home because there was nothing they could do as the tumour was growing into his brain. It is such a sad, sad place and my heart is heavy.

Letter to Sophie, Day 113, Friday 9 April 2004
We left you in the capable hands of Catherine this morning, as we were heading home with Mitchell to complete our *60 Minutes* interview. Grandma Joy took Mitchell with Dee and Carol [friends from New Zealand] down to Clontarf for

a picnic and swim. The *60 Minutes* team have been really easy to work with. We gave the interviews because we wanted to highlight burns injuries and to thank the public for their amazing support. We have been privileged to be the recipients of such goodwill and it is ongoing to this day, seventeen weeks after the accident.

Beckie is your daytime nurse, which is lovely. Nana and Nanu, Manuel and Carmen came to visit, and Lyn was with you as well. When your head is looking left, you don't have much mobility in your neck, so we will have to do more head turns and, when you are sleeping prone overnight, have you with your head turned left at all times.

Carolyn's journal, Day 113, Friday 9 April 2004
Soph had a stable night but her temperature peaked at 39.6 degrees. We left her at 10 am, as we were to be interviewed by *60 Minutes*. We tried to be frank and honest. It was sort of normal being at home with Mitchell and Ron and in the car driving back. We headed back to hospital and smiling Dave was there to greet us for coffee and a laugh.

Letter to Sophie, Day 114, Saturday 10 April 2004
Ron called at 10 am to say you were having a dressing change. I came up to be with Mitchell, and he and I did puzzles. Dr Andy was pleased with the graft – fragile but looking at this stage like a ninety- to ninety-five-per-cent take. Your grafts are being treated open, so you have Jelonet on the grafted sites – it looks raw and exposed but Dr Andy and Dr Peter are pleased, so this is a good thing!

Beckie is your nurse again today and she is lovely with you, so gentle and kind and encouraging. John and Katrina arrived and looked after Mitchell for a bit, until you were settled. Dad then took Mitchell to the Easter Show, which he had been looking forward to for some time. Your temperature spiked today at forty degrees, so you have been put back onto the three antibiotics you have been on before for staph and *Pseudomonas*.

We play music and rainbow stories for you. Your eyes are swollen from being prone, so you cannot see. Because you are so immobile, music and stories are about all we can do for you, except for special oils to smell and, when you wake, a story or two. Today, a lady brought handmade angels to you, for Lilly and Molly and for each of the injured children of the Roundhouse; they are beautiful. Beckie thinks you are amazingly tolerant for everything you've been through – you are BRAVE!

Carolyn's journal, Day 114, Saturday 10 April 2004
Today heralds a dressing change, bed change and ventilation-tube re-taping, which takes about three hours. The re-taping of the tube requires Sophie to be rolled at forty-five degrees, with Andy, two doctors and two nurses present. This will have to be done daily. Sophie is being nursed prone and uncovered, with Jelonet only over her back and head. I keep looking at her photo to remind myself of the real Sophie – her spirit is so strong to endure what she is now. I hope she has no memory of this.

Ron's journal, Day 114, Saturday 10 April 2004
Still taking antidepressants at the moment and still feel that's what I need to do. I've been thinking a lot about what Sophie's gone through and I think I've been concentrating so much on what Sophie hasn't got any more – she hasn't got her feet, she hasn't got her toes, she hasn't got the fingers of her right hand, her right ear, a lot of muscle tissue. She probably hasn't got a childhood any more; I think that's been robbed from her. And I've realised that I've been concentrating so much on that – the things that she hasn't got – instead of concentrating on what

we have got, the fact that we still have our family, we still have Sophie and Mitchell. Hopefully, everything will be all right and we will all be together again. I think this is probably the turnaround in my health and in being able to deal with the whole situation.

Letter to Sophie, Day 115, Sunday 11 April 2004
I spent a lot of today reading research pages that our friend, Jo Hansen, found through her Google searches; I feel inspired to continue the research into your ongoing care. You have been blessed with wonderful support. The information is detailed and thorough. I feel destiny will mean we all benefit from the information gathered.

Today is Easter Sunday and you have a great big fluffy bunny sitting on a chair. The girls in Clubbe Ward wanted you to know the Easter bunny had been to you, so they sent it upstairs. Mitchell had a lovely Easter-egg hunt and went happily off with Mary on the JetCat to Luna Park. Dee and Carol came, and we sat out in the gardens – the weather has cooled down enough to do that without getting too hot. Despite the fact that your dressings are uncovered, you spiked today at thirty-nine degrees. You are back on the Medaz, after being weaned off it overnight, because you became agitated after a dressing change where Bactigrass was used. We are not sure why it was used, but this is the difference between being in PICU and the greater control we have in the Burns ward. You have been much more settled this afternoon and evening. We play classical music and your rainbow-story CD. I hope it makes you feel less alone – I love you.

Carolyn's journal, Day 115, Sunday 11 April 2004
Sophie had a dressing change and became quite unsettled. Bactigrass was used, as the tummy had a fair amount of pus,

and we think this contributed to the agitation. Ron went to get scarlet red from the Burns ward. Peter Hayward came to check on Sophie and it appears that about eighty per cent of the grafts have taken.

It is difficult to sit and see your beautiful child endure lying prone, intubated, totally exposed and raw. Rationally, we know it is ultimately for her benefit, but her injuries are a cruel reminder – being so 'in your face'. While the intense pain has dulled due to the exposure to such extreme care requirements, the emotional toll wrenches at your heart every minute.

Dee and Carol visited, which was lovely. I spoke of how proud I was of Mitchell and how he, through this, has grown up (rather forcefully – lost some innocence) but has had the benefit of care from friends (as well as extended family). In a rather wonderful way, he counts our friends as his, and thankfully they are delighted to be involved in his and Sophie's care. I only hope it continues, because I see a lot of good coming from this.

Beckie told us that Peter is moving away from Burns, though he will still follow Sophie's case. I know he was devastated when we lost seventy per cent of the head grafts – Andy told us this. I have decided I will research, research, research to give Sophie the best for her care requirements. Sometimes, I still think that this is all just a ghastly dream and that my precious one is still her happy self. My heart aches for us to be back at that place where we felt so blessed to be together as a family.

Letter to Sophie, Day 116, Monday 12 April 2004
My beautiful daughter, how I love you and miss you. These last four days with you intubated and unable to communicate other than nodding your head have been lonely. I want to have you back in the Burns ward so I can sit behind you in bed, play with you, read you stories and sing songs with you. Tomorrow, you

may be extubated; you will certainly have a dressing change and be turned over. Today, scarlet red was placed on your grafted sites but you still remain exposed. We play more upbeat music during the day for you, like the Wiggles, and stories for you during your dressing changes. Your lilac pillow is ever present and your room is a calm, peaceful haven.

I am reading a story called *Waking the Tiger* [by Peter Levine, about healing past traumas], which I hope will help with your overall healing. I've had a quiet night, cleaning some of your toys and enjoying some rare solitude. At times, I feel there is too much to do in a day. I need to block out time to get some things ticked off my list – or at least delegate them. We shall travel a wonderful path together; you will never be alone and your shining spirit will carry you miles.

Carolyn's journal, Day 116, Monday 12 April 2004
Today, Amy and I changed Sophie's arm and leg dressings and put scarlet red on her back. Although John [Delezio] took Mitchell to the Starlight Room [a doctor-free zone with games, craft and entertainment for children in hospital], I suspect Mitchell saw some of Sophie exposed today. Mum came over and I thought it important for her to see Sophie's wounds, as she may be helping with her dressings in future.

Ron and Mitchell walked back from Parramatta and played in the park. Then they headed home this afternoon to swim in our neighbours' new pool. I stayed in Sophie's room reading till eight. I feel I need a day to myself tomorrow, although I think they will do a dressing change and keep Sophie prone. They may want her back in the ward tomorrow night. I hope I can have one more decent sleep. I read a story about a wife as caregiver to her husband who dies after twelve months in her care and I can relate to her struggle; it made me cry.

Letter to Sophie, Day 117, Tuesday 13 April 2004
This morning, your dressings were placed on your back in anticipation of you being turned supine [face upwards, lying on the back]. It was a happy moment to see you turned, your face very swollen but beautiful. You had a lot of medication for your dressing change, which has kept you pretty still this afternoon. Cheri put the plaster casts on and did physio with you. The ladies in the volunteer room gave me a box of CDs and tapes, so you had a greater selection. Beth sat with you today, as we were being interviewed by *Woman's Day*; it was lovely to have her sitting holding your hand and selecting music for you. *60 Minutes* and the *Woman's Day* article will have account details so funds can be channelled to the Burns Unit at Westmead, which we hope will build a legacy so other people can benefit from the things we have learnt and seen while we have been here.

Carolyn's journal, Day 117, Tuesday 13 April 2004
A happy day, as Sophie is turned. Sophie is mouthing 'water', as she has been fasted since 4 am in anticipation of extubation, which has now been postponed till tomorrow. It is now 5 pm, so feeds are going back on. Louise knows her needs well; she always has the lavender pillow ready and music or stories playing. Sophie has opened one eye, as the swelling has gone down. She has just a few fingers poking out of the top of her plaster cast and I kiss them and her forehead.

Ron's journal, Day 117, Tuesday 13 April 2004
Came up to Sophie's room to find all of her recent grafts were very mucky. Andy came in and was equally disturbed, until he started wiping the creamy top off the grafts. They still looked okay. Andy cleaned all of the grafts and wanted to put Jelonet dressings on again. I talked him into using scarlet red again, due to its antibacterial nature. We also discussed with Dr David

[Murrell] that we will halve the Medazolan around midnight tonight and they would change it to diazepam later. If this did not work, then they would go back to Medazolan.

Letter to Sophie, Day 118, Wednesday 14 April 2004
Tonight, it's hard to get into the routines we had in the Burns ward previously. Louise is your nurse today; she has worked with you a lot in the past and does reiki. Therese came down today to harmonise you. The process works on balancing your chakra and your electromagnetic fields. Therese was able to harmonise me too and I felt wonderful as a result – energised.

You're extubated at around midday and monitored all afternoon, and everyone is very pleased with your progress. Grandma Joy and Beth sit in with you while Dad and I are in a meeting with your medical team. We need to get more mobility in your neck when you are prone, so you go to sleep with your right side down.

Carolyn's journal, Day 118, Wednesday 14 April 2004
Extubated at last and moved to Burns Unit. The care received in PICU is wonderful; it would be great to have that on the Burns ward, but we are back to a very hands-on approach. Which is fine – just a matter of readjusting again. These are the differences: we have to call the shots and ask for things to be done other than meds administered. It was difficult getting Sophie into position, particularly her head. At the meeting today, we were advised that Sophie will not have the muscle strength to hold her right arm up above her head. Ninety degrees will be manageable.

Letter to Sophie, Day 119, Thursday 15 April 2004

I have come home for the night to pick up Mitchell. We took Zach's birthday present to him as the baby is due today, so we may not see them at hospital for a while. We had pizza and pasta, and Zach enjoyed his toolset. I sat down and turned the TV on to the *Footy Show* to see 'The Birdman Competition' held in Manly, in aid of the Molly Wood and Sophie Delezio Trust Fund. Matty Johns was there and did a great job entertaining the crowd.

This morning, you slept till 9.30 am. We had you sitting and reacquainting yourself with your toys, books, puzzles and presents. You slept 11.30 am–12.30 pm, when it was dressing-change time. It was a full dressing change in the shower bath. You kicked your legs like you were swimming. Everyone is happy with the way your skin is healing. I can't help but feel you are ready for rehab. If it had been possible, I'm sure you would be trying to get mobile, so we will concentrate on sitting you up and getting you in your chair. You have two less pumps attached to your bed, which could be the boost we need in our efforts to get you mobile.

chapter eleven
Sophie's legs

With each month that passes, Sophie is a little older and a little more aware of her injuries, beyond the immediate pain. As she starts to ask questions about her hands and legs, Ron and Carolyn see that the time has come to start to talk to Sophie about what has happened to her. It is a conversation that no parents can imagine having with their child, but there is no avoiding it.

At last, Sophie can start to explore the world outside the ward, pushed in her wheelchair in the lush gardens that surround the Children's Hospital at Westmead. Whenever Sophie goes for a walk, she has to be hooked up to a portable drip filled with morphine. It's a restricted drug, so a nurse needs to go with her each and every time.

Sophie now has to undergo just one more graft to achieve full coverage of skin. It's far from the end of grafting for her, though: throughout her childhood and adolescence, she will need a series of operations. Her damaged skin will grow more slowly than it needs to, so her doctors will need to do 'contracture releases' to allow her bones to grow unimpeded.

Letter to Sophie, Day 120, Friday 16 April 2004
Mitchell and I arrived at 11.15 after having a look at a house that may be suitable for us long-term. Sandra saw Mitchell and he raised a few things about being really scared when you were up at PICU. It made him really uncomfortable that we didn't want him in your room, but that was because when your dressings were open your skin was still quite raw.

He played with you this afternoon and you laughed together. You didn't want to share your crayons with him, though, and got quite upset when he could do drawings and you couldn't because you had your plaster cast on. You were asleep when Lisa came to play, so she did some craft with Mitchell instead; I really hope that you can do some playing in the shop/cooking/dough tomorrow. It's Molly's birthday party and Mitchell will go. You had soup and pasta and a little chicken tonight. Magic Maree came and sprinkled fairy dust on you. Dee and Carol visited on their way back from Canberra and the South Coast. We will have to start the bedtime routine a little earlier each night to get you into bed at a reasonable hour: 10 pm is too late!

Carolyn's journal, Day 120, Friday 16 April 2004
A busy morning getting Mitchell organised and out of the house by 9.30 to view Seaforth Crescent with [real-estate agent] Erica. The land would suit us very well – it's big enough for us to build a home, complete with swimming pool for hydrotherapy; we shall see if it is possible.

Mitchell is getting quite clingy with me at the moment. I'll take him to the movies on Sunday. *60 Minutes* wanted an extra shoot with photos and they interviewed the doctors today. *Woman's Day* came to finish their photo shoot – it felt more staged than the filming, where we just got on and did what we would be doing anyway. Soph had a sleepy morning, then we talked and played together. She slept for an hour and then we went for a walk outside in the wheelchair – it is much easier without the additional monitors. We had feeds off, so only one pump. Sophie enjoyed it but got a bit hot.

Letter to Sophie, Day 121, Saturday 17 April 2004
You slept prone till 10.30. That's thirteen hours – well done. You did very well in your full dressing change; it took an hour and a half. Andy wants it every two days. We'll have to see how you manage; we don't want you to be so tired that you don't want to do anything during the day. You had Karen visit from Prague and Lee, Linda, Wayne and Lillie as well as Carolyn, James and Charlotte. Your temperature got up to 38.5 today, the hottest it's been for two days. Your catheter is leaking, so we will see what Andy suggests we do about this tomorrow. You told me you were burnt in a fire today when you were watching a Wiggles video with some firefighters on it. You also asked what they were wearing, particularly the scarf over their head. When I said they wear that so their head doesn't get burnt, you said, 'I didn't.' Later that night, I asked how you knew you were burnt in a fire and you just looked at me and didn't say anything.

Carolyn's journal, Day 121, Saturday 17 April 2004
Sophie watched the Wiggles video on New York firefighters and she started asking questions. Then we saw a picture of a fireman putting out a fire and she said, 'I was in a fire and got burnt but the doctors and nurses, Mummy and Daddy are helping me to get well.' I was lost for words, so I added, 'And Mitchell, all your friends and some people you don't even know are helping you get better by sending you their love.'

Carolyn and James and Charlotte visited and brought fruit. Thank goodness – I keep feeling I am missing fruit and veg.

Sophie's legs

Letter to Sophie, Day 122, Sunday 18 April 2004
Mitchell and I went to the movies to see *The Cat in the Hat*; he really wanted to see you afterwards but you were asleep. I arrived and gave you a great big kiss. You slept till 2.30, when Tracey, Jo, Fleur and Georgia [friends] arrived with a video for your birthday present. It has all your favourite things on it, even the Wiggles singing 'Happy Birthday'. You smiled a lot during it, which was lovely to see.

We put you in your chair and you played chasing with Mitchell, with Daddy pushing. You laughed and smiled again. Your appetite is improving: nuts, ham, chicken-noodle soup, spaghetti, mince and chips, all in very small amounts. Yesterday, you drank some of Dad's tomato juice. With your catheter out, you are doing well. You even said to me, 'I need a new nappy.' You were singing Dorothy songs this evening, and I got your Dorothy and Jeff dolls to sing along – this made you laugh. Daddy and Mitchell rang, and we all sent each other rainbows.

Carolyn's journal, Day 122, Sunday 18 April 2004
Tracey et al. brought by a beautiful birthday video made specially for Sophie. It's wonderful: people from the zoo, animations and the Wiggles. Dee and Carol came over too and said farewell before they head back to New Zealand early tomorrow – it was lovely having them here and Carol was very good with Mitchell. Grandma Joy came too. Sophie reached 38.2 degrees today. Movements very limited and she complains of being hurt, saying 'you hurt me' a lot. Mitchell is getting quite clingy, so I agreed to go home next Wednesday afternoon and read him a story at day care.

Letter to Sophie, Day 123, Monday 19 April 2004
Today was a busy day, with meeting the new registrar on the

ward and speaking to Andy about your temperature spikes. Linda came with Elysa and Lillie to visit – you were singing songs and having stories. Daddy and I met Nadia to discuss your wheelchairs, then we met with the fund-raising department to make sure funds are properly distributed to the Burns ward. I met with Sandra about an ongoing strategy with you in relation to your growing awareness of why you are in hospital. We are at present trying to get a urine sample, which doesn't want to come. The day simply disappeared and I didn't even get outside. You are a brave little girl and everyone is amazed at how well you are coping with your dressing changes and physio exercises. We aim to get you outside more and sitting in your chair. Your appetite is small but you are getting a good variety of meals.

Carolyn's journal, Day 123, Monday 19 April 2004
Exhausting – drained and down. These days are when you feel the long journey ahead. Sophie had temps overnight, so I woke anxious to get it sorted. Spoke with the pain-team doctor about reducing pain med so that we can get the line out at the appropriate time. I spoke to the Infectious Diseases doctor about starting antibiotics rather than waiting for blood results. Andy came to dressing change and agreed we start asap. Line looks okay. Attended dressing change – breakdown of skin on left leg, hypergranulation and *Pseudomonas* under right arm. I get stressed when they are short staffed. No one knew what pain meds to do. Two is not enough – it seemed messy, so I will take control.

Letter to Sophie, Day 124, Tuesday 20 April 2004
Sleep till 10 am, then plaster casts off and bloods taken – nappy change and into the chair for 11 am. Lisa arranged the table so you could paint, draw and play with dough. Louise [Palmer] came

when you were watching *The Lion King* and you slept for forty-five minutes before being woken by nursing staff needing to fix monitors, fluids, milk and antibiotics, which had crystallised in the pump. Louise stayed with you while Daddy and I proofed the *Woman's Day* article. You were watching your Sophie birthday video, which you love to see over and over again.

Louise, Linda and Beth came out this evening for mah-jong. We didn't play – instead, we came in to see you because you had woken at 8.30. We gave you pizza and you were very excited, having friends in your room. It took a while to settle you once you were prone and throughout the night you had constant sleep disruption because of monitors beeping, meds being given, stats monitored, temperature taken. Then, because broken sleep increases your pain awareness, you needed boluses to put you back to sleep. Your chin is being rubbed on your mattress, so we will have to put something soft over it – it does mean, though, you are turning your head to make yourself more comfortable.

When you get grumpy, you have taken to spitting, which is not nice. When you are happy, you will doze on your bed with your legs and arms going, usually to the Wiggles.

Letter to Sophie, Day 125, Wednesday 21 April 2004
A tough night, with monitors going off. You wake whenever the nurses are in the room. You sleep till your dressing change in the morning. It finishes at 12.30 pm and we catch up with the Wood family outside for some shots with *60 Minutes*. Grandma Joy stays with you but you sleep pretty much all afternoon. Dad and I go straight to our medic meeting, where I address a number of issues on my 'list'. Andy suggested padded earmuffs for you, so you can sleep through anything.

I treated myself to a massage, then checked in on you – you

were still asleep at 4.30 pm. Grandma, Mitchell and I headed home for the evening. I put Mitchell to bed for 8.30; he slept on the way home from hospital. I sat with Ma after dinner and we had a chat. It's really nice and comfortable being at home, and I can't wait to bring you home too! You will need to find a way of moving around rooms and I have no doubt you will rise to every challenge ahead of you. I believe you are an inspiration and will be a great teacher to many. You have already taught me so much in your three years: decisiveness, strength, courage, bravery, love, trust, openness, faith.

Carolyn's journal, Day 125, Wednesday 21 April 2004
One more graft to go, most likely next Thursday. Soph will be going home with staples – she has as many as twelve in her chest that we haven't even seen. They will, however, remove as many as they can next theatre.

Letter to Sophie, Day 126, Thursday 22 April 2004
I spent today at home with Mitchell. Grandma Joy had arranged for friends to play: Mischa, Byron, Taylor and Michael. Melissa, Jessica and Christopher came too, and Melissa suggested that Jessica come and play with you, which was lovely of her. She is going to arrange for the mobile zoo to come to the ward for you, Sophie.

You talked to Dad about your legs being hurt in a fire last night and today he felt the opportunity presented itself to talk to you about your legs. Mary and Sandra were with him when he told you that because your legs had been burnt so badly the doctors couldn't save them and that you would get new legs and they would be fast. Daddy cried after he told you.

We want to have the firefighter who lifted you from under the car visit you, if he agrees. It is now time to piece the puzzle together for you so you have a clear understanding. The one thing that is the most important is that you know we love you unconditionally and will help you in any way we can.

Carolyn's journal, Day 126, Thursday 22 April 2004
I spent the day with Mitchell till 5 pm. Today, Ron rang and said he had told Sophie about her legs. It brought it home in leaps and bounds. I cried when I was at home – it is all too raw still. Mitchell had some friends over. I spoke with all their mothers and I felt drained driving back to hospital.

Letter to Sophie, Day 127, Friday 23 April 2004
Daddy was with you for a dressing change while I spent some time with Mitchell and Sandra. We put you in your chair and went outside for finger-painting. Your infections seem to have stabilised and your morphine has been reduced. You managed your dressing change well and seemed happy and comfortable this afternoon with the lower morphine rate. More Wiggles Band-Aids were purchased – they have to be purple. Because your arms are in plaster casts, we cannot use your hands for games but I'm hoping to do some play with puzzles over the weekend. We will certainly get you out in the chair in the evenings; the days are still too warm. You want to have dinner outside – maybe tomorrow.

Letter to Sophie, Day 128, Saturday 24 April 2004
A sunny, happy day for you today, probably your best. Mitchell arranged a picnic for you. He wrote 'picnic' on your outside door. We talked about the food that was needed and Mitchell arranged all the chairs. Katrina was with us all day and stayed

with you while we went for a walk with Mitchell. Catherine and Antoni came for the picnic and we played chasing with Mitchell and Antoni. You have been singing songs today. We played with some puzzles and Mitchell was happy to spend the large part of the day with us all in your room. You were wearing a neck brace, which gives you a greater range of movement for your neck.

Today, we removed the nasal prongs and you did really well without your oxygen, so we will keep it off. I have not increased your morphine overnight at this stage, so we'll see how you manage that. We gave you some prosthetic limbs to look at today and you said, 'Now I can walk!' We said, 'You're tall,' and you said, 'I bigger than Mitchell.' He got a bit concerned about that. I gave you a hug today and you said, 'I do it,' and gave me the most beautiful hug back by lifting your arm and attempting to give me a big hug – it melted my heart.

Letter to Sophie, Day 129, Sunday 25 April 2004
This morning, we had you sitting in your chair watching videos with Mitchell. When Catherine and Antoni came, we went outside and played with puzzles. You were in your chair for three hours, then bed for a sleep.

Sister Bridget came over; so did Mandy and her new beau, a very good-looking South American. We watched your 'Sophie is three' video again and then played with musical instruments and more puzzles. You shared, unprompted, your Easter eggs in your pink handbag with Dad, Mandy and her friend and Mitchell. You were a bit tired today but we still had some beautiful moments. I can't wait till we can take you for walks outside the ward. We visited the Careflight helipad, and the helicopter pilots invited Mitchell and Antoni on board. I think I'll sit behind you tomorrow and we can do stuff together.

Carolyn's journal, Day 129, Sunday 25 April 2004
Last night, Sophie was unsettled. She wanted to go onto her back at 4 am. She did one big vomit, slept till 9 am, then we got her into the chair. I gave Sophie a hug and she said, 'I cuddle you, Mum.' It melts my heart. Mitchell massaged Sophie's tummy with the massager tonight and is interacting more with her.

Letter to Sophie, Day 130, Monday 26 April 2004
A cheery smile when I arrived in your room this morning. Dad wasn't feeling well and he was going to take Mitchell to the water slides at Manly to attend a fund-raiser for you and Molly. Beth took Max and they were meeting other friends there, so Mitchell and Dad were home this afternoon. Nanu rang up as he saw the article in *Woman's Day* and was very pleased; he has bought extra to send to Malta.

Nurse Dianne came into the parents' room, where I was having a cup of tea while you slept, to say you were dreaming and your heartbeats dropped to ninety-six per minute – the lowest today I saw was a hundred and fourteen, so you are doing very well. I sat behind you and we watched *Monsters Inc*. Then Grandma and I took you for your first walk outside the ward: down to the aviary and children's garden fountain. You didn't want to go back inside but the morphine pump ran out of batteries. Before our walk, we were having afternoon tea outside your room and you wanted to chase the birds: your little legs were running to chase them. You are just too beautiful. I'm so proud of you.

Letter to Sophie, Day 131, Tuesday 27 April 2004
We had you painting today on your yellow table in your

tumble-form chair on your bed. We then tested a new upright chair and will try to have you in it for ten minutes tomorrow. We took you outside to chase birds in your wheelchair. Dr Peter and Dr Andy came to visit and are pleased with your progress. The graft was scheduled for Thursday, with a suggestion of being able to take your central line and your NG tube out as soon as possible after that. You will have to have a catheter in after this op, as your graft/donor sites are too close to your bottom and lower abdomen.

You were saying 'shush shush shush' tonight; we asked what that was and you said it's the noise fire makes. Then you said fire is hot. You were singing a bit to Captain Starlight this morning and were happy and chatty this afternoon. You built some blocks and made a tower three blocks high. Tonight, we had to use your 'funky chick' pillow and you are still not asleep, happily kicking your legs about while lying prone.

Carolyn's journal, Day 131, Tuesday 27 April 2004
Sophie managed having both her arms on the yellow table and did great finger-painting. She also trialled her new chair and managed that well, surprising Jo, Sarah [Clubbe Ward nurse] and Louise. Lee and Mark came over to visit, and Sophie asked Mark to find her a swimming video. Parramatta Police dropped in a big bear and Mary Wilson wanted to know if Sophie needed a new teddy; I suggested instead she knit her a new cardy, and she was thrilled.

Letter to Sophie, Day 132, Wednesday 28 April 2004
A very wakeful night, so a new mattress has been designed: a flat piece of foam and a separate pillow. You managed your dressing change very well; I carried you there on my shoulders and you saw Molly going in for her bath [as an outpatient]

at the same time. You kissed my shoulders on the way back to the room. Lyn came back from Bali and brought an orange fairy dress for you and a Spiderman outfit for Mitchell. You manage the bath beautifully and have new stockings/pantyhose on your legs. Catherine and Antoni come, and Lee and Mark with a DVD from Ian Thorpe of his swimming. 'Sophie is very chatty today,' said Lyn. You also had very short sleeps but that allowed us to put you on your new mattress at 8.30 pm. So we will see how this goes overnight: hopefully, a better sleep for all.

We are going for a walk outside tomorrow before your operation, which will be the second last before your central line comes out. The one tomorrow will be your last for full coverage and, after close to twenty weeks, your beautiful body will be able to heal. My precious miracle.

Carolyn's journal, Day 132, Wednesday 28 April 2004
A shocking sleep but a great dressing change on our return. From that, I went to review the *60 Minutes* tape; it got the thumbs-up. It was then time for a massage and Zen harmonising, followed by the burns meeting, then back to the room. Sophie said in the bath today, 'Tigger is at Mitchell's house.' I said, 'Your house, too,' and Sophie said, 'No, Mitchell's house.' Andy mentioned a contracture release in a couple of weeks, then removal of the line and NG tube. We are on the homeward track.

Letter to Sophie, Day 133, Thursday 29 April 2004
A great sleep with the new mattress – just a few wakeful periods. We decided to go for a walk early and we needed some clothes for the 'big walk' so I went to the volunteers' shop and they found a dress and nightie for you. With a bandanna on,

you looked stunning. One of the nurses, Merly, took us to the aviary and Chinese garden. We said 'hi' to the volunteers and to Debbie, whose son suffered cancer and had amputations. Physio trialled you in the new chair and thought ten minutes would be good but you made it for one hour – well done! We thought you were going to theatre so let you watch *Monsters Inc*. Dad had a cuddle in bed, with you sitting on his lap. Maree came over in the afternoon all dressed in pink and kept you entertained while I caught up with Jan. Mary played with Mitchell this afternoon and brought him in with pizzas.

Carolyn's journal, Day 133, Thursday 29 April 2004
I managed to get to t'ai chi. Then physio arranged the new chair in the wheelchair and took off plasters. In the chair at 9.45 and we left at 10 am for a walk. We waited for theatre booked for 1.30 but an emergency came in so we didn't go. Sophie was asleep at 6.30 pm, so it will be interesting to see how her night goes. Ron's on duty. Sophie had a happy, chatty day and was really entertaining. A lady rang today and said, 'You don't know me but I'm arranging a fund-raiser for the girls through Dundas Rugby Club.' The community support is amazing.

Letter to Sophie, Day 134, Friday 30 April 2004
This morning, you had a bath with no nitrous oxide – no mask. Fantastic. Everyone thought you did really well. Lyn came and painted your nails, then you had a big sleep while Dad did some work. You were busy singing 'Arabella Miller' all evening and, although happy, complained of a sore bottom. I think you have been sitting on that bed too long – we will have to work on your mobility and arrange for someone to take you for a walk on Saturday and Sunday. I'll see if we can be off IV morphine for half an hour so we can go for a walk without nurses.

Carolyn's journal, Day 134, Friday 30 April 2004
The rural firefighters came in and Sophie and Mitchell met them. Mitch and I went to the Starlight Room and played bingo. Took Mitch back to the room for bath time and another video while Ron and I did the switch. A long discussion with David Murrell and the pain fellow with both Ron and myself leaves us with the impression it could be less than three weeks before we are out of hospital.

chapter twelve
days of progress

The response to the 60 Minutes *story on Sophie and Molly is overwhelming. Both families are flooded with letters, calls and messages from complete strangers expressing their support and their thanks for the inspiration they felt in seeing these young girls overcoming such adversity.*

Ron and Carolyn themselves are still learning about Sophie's accident. In the immediate aftermath of the Roundhouse fire, all of their energies went into keeping Sophie alive. They never received a full account of what had happened in the childcare centre that day. So that they can be prepared to tell Sophie about it, they must now find out more about the events that threatened their little girl's life. It is a quest that renews the sadness they both feel.

As Sophie is able to leave her room more and explore the world beyond the hospital, going home will soon be a reality.

Letter to Sophie, Day 135, Saturday 1 May 2004
What a great day! I stayed in bed as well till 9.45 am. Ron went home to look at our house, which is being rendered. I arranged to have you off morphine for an hour while John and Katrina helped rearrange your room with the shelves they brought so we can display all your toys to play with. Gracie [another patient] and her family – Felicity, Clare, Margaret and Graham – arrived, and you and Mitchell painted Gracie's toenails on her prosthetic legs. They are a wonderful family and Gracie left some special Ugg boots for you and a beautiful orange blanket. When they left, we went inside and Stephanie, your nurse, found us a mat. We put your new blanket down and you sat on my knee. You saw all your toys and wanted to play with lots, until you said you wanted to go back to bed. You promptly fell asleep at 6.30 pm. Daddy is sleeping in with you tonight, so I hope you are good for him!

Carolyn's journal, Day 135, Saturday 1 May 2004
I stayed in bed till 9.45 am, catching half-hour intervals from 5 am. The night nurses can be loud and clumsy and clearly have no idea how difficult it is to sleep with them thumping around. If Sophie stirred when the light went on, one of them would ask, 'What's the matter, Sophie?' and try to engage her in talking when all she wanted to do was sleep. She also leaves her room door open and there were lots of crying babies last night. At 12.30 pm, Ron arrived back and we went for a walk with no pumps. Sophie went to the Starlight Room, aviary and Chinese garden. All in all, a great day of progress.

Letter to Sophie, Day 136, Sunday 2 May 2004
I have just watched the *60 Minutes* story. We had agreed that our principal aims in doing the story were to 1) thank everyone for their support, 2) tell the story that all families of seriously ill

children face in living in hospital, and 3) educate the public on the treatment of burns and continuing treatment requirements over the years. We all wanted something you would be proud of in the future. Daddy is online to answer any questions and we were asking for donations for the Burns ward. There were five hundred emailed questions and hundreds of letters of support. Some commented that they found the story inspirational, so if it changes someone's life for the better then I'm pleased. We wanted something good to come from the tragedy. We had turned you prone at 7 pm but while I was in the parents' room you did a big poo and vomit. Pam [Cheung] and Margaret [Maroney, Clubbe Ward nurses] changed you while *60 Minutes* was on. You stopped crying and said, 'There's Mummy. There's Sophie [Fofie]. There's Daddy. There's Mitchell.'

Carolyn's journal, Day 136, Sunday 2 May 2004
Today, we went for a long walk to the Starlight Room, Chinese gardens, aviary and past the children's garden. Sophie was a little bit quiet for this walk, although she enjoyed it. Sophie was back in bed by 3.30 pm and asleep by four. I'm watching *60 Minutes* and I cry. We will watch a video of the show together with Mitchell.

Letter to Sophie, Day 137, Monday 3 May 2004
I received a call from a woman called Therese, in Perth. She saw *60 Minutes* and was praying for you, Sophie, and knows God will look after you and take care of you. Another lady, from Adelaide, wants to make you some clothes. You received more letters and cards today. You went to surgery for the last time to be covered today and Dr Andy said you went very well. This leaves only one operation in a fortnight's time to release your contractures and then we are homeward bound, assuming your meds are okay.

days of progress

You came back to the ward after the op and you were quite unsettled. You needed the maximum of all your meds to settle you and there was nothing more I could do, so I went to sleep in the parents' room for a couple of hours. Pam, a wonderful nurse with ten years of experience with burns patients, is with you and I know you are in the best hands. It's 12.30 am; I'll head back to the room to check on you before calling it a night. *60 Minutes* was overwhelmed with calls of support for you. I love you!

Carolyn's journal, Day 137, Monday 3 May 2004
I'm bloody angry. Sophie came back from theatre without low-dose ketamine – she was thrashing about from 6.30 to 8 pm, settled from 8 to 10 pm and has been thrashing around since then. Sophie's bed is not operating properly and she will not be able to go prone because of it. Her thrashing will prevent her splints going on. If she keeps those grafts, I will be amazed. 'Knee hurting, shoulder hurting, arm hurting, hips hurting, head hurting.' Can't find file with ketamine infusion noted. Anaesthetic registrar came down. Sophie screamed from 10 to 12 am, kicked and twisted about.

Letter to Sophie, Day 138, Tuesday 4 May 2004
Today, you slept. Your ketamine was added at 11 pm and you slept from 1 to 4 am, woke for five minutes and slept again. I stayed with you on and off all morning as you slept till 11 am. You slept from 1 to 4 pm, when we watched videos with Dad. You were asleep by 8 pm.

We are having discussions about us going home. At the latest, it will be the end of June – that's around seven weeks! You will be able to swim when your skin has healed. You are lying on your mattress tonight saying mask, goggles, swimsuit, bubbles, Barbie board – obviously very excited about it all.

Your donor sites for this last graft are your buttocks and lower abdomen, so we have a catheter in because we didn't want your donor site to sting any more than it does. I have popped out of the room because you have rung the kitchen and asked for pizza. You keep asking me to check with them to see if it is ready yet. The difficulty is the kitchen isn't open and even if we had pizza you wouldn't eat more than a mouthful anyway. Your personality still shines through all and I'm proud of you.

Letter to Sophie, Day 139, Wednesday 5 May 2004
We have lovely playtime in your special seat and little yellow table. You chose all the toys, puzzles and drawings and managed an hour and a quarter before your back got sore. You are holding your head even better than on Monday. Lyn brought you McDonald's, which you said you would eat 'later'. I went shopping for you today so that you have something to wear; I'll be remodelling all sorts of things in the future, I think. You are happy and chatty, and although you get frustrated when things don't quite work how you like them, you don't let it bother you for long. I keep saying to you 'not to worry, Sophie, we'll find a way'.

Letter to Sophie, Day 140, Thursday 6 May 2004
Mary came and spent the day with us, which was great; she entertained both you and Mitchell. You had X-rays on both legs to check them and really enjoyed being out and about. You didn't want to go back to your bed. You have not been sleeping that well and you don't have much upper-body strength. You sat in your new chair and yellow table but after ten minutes you

had your head on the table, unable to support it even with the collar. Your arms are plastered at the elbow and at the wrists, so you have two separate casts on, which makes movement difficult and may be the reason you do not settle easily overnight. We try all sorts of pain regimes to make you more comfortable. It is hard for all of us because we are learning along the way, along with the doctors and nurses.

Carolyn's journal, Day 140, Thursday 6 May 2004

The day disappeared. Mary arrived, as did Ron and Mitchell at lunchtime. We had dinner at the restaurant upstairs for the first time since being here. I discussed some business matters with Mary and took Mitchell to bed at 9.30 – too late!

Letter to Sophie, Day 141, Friday 7 May 2004

Vomiting today, although no apparent reason. You want your nappy off tonight and wiggle your bottom around on your new mattress. An exciting day, because you met with Charli from Hi-5 and Paul Francis, who runs the Humpty Dumpty Foundation. Daddy is going to be a guest speaker for them. You were harmonised today as well.

This morning, we went for walks to the aviary and fish pond and around the gardens. You were given lots of mail today – some lovely gifts and wonderful letters, cards and messages of support. We are very privileged, because lots of long-term families are here and live miles away with no support.

You are quite unsettled tonight and I just don't know how to make you comfortable, so I give you a cuddle and say a prayer. We have tried a dozen different pillows and none seems to work satisfactorily, so tiredness will just take over and you will settle in time. I love you and feel for you.

Carolyn's journal, Day 141, Friday 7 May 2004
Mitchell and I stayed in the room till just after 10.30 am – we slept in the sofa bed last night. It was a restful sleep, except Mitchell woke at 7.30 am. I sorted gifts and letters and tidied the room. It is looking even more likely that we will be going home by early June. Mitchell and Soph watched DVDs on Sophie's bed. It was the first time Mitchell would sit on it. Dr Peter called by to 'pay his respects' – he is a special man. I'm on 'Sophie night' tonight, with special mattress mark four.

Letter to Sophie, Day 142, Saturday 8 May 2004
Sophie, you eventually settled at 1 am last night, then you slept till 11 am. We had you up in your chair from midday till 6.30 pm, which was a great effort. We went for a couple of walks around the hospital with Katrina and [Minister for Health] Tony Abbott. We saw all the artwork down one ward and went to the aviary again.

Carolyn and Charlotte came to play, and Mitchell and you were very excited. We had you in your chair outside your room playing marbles, painting, chasing Mitchell and finding balls. It was a pleasant autumn afternoon, with the leaves on the crepe myrtle turning orange. You were sweating a lot today, despite the mild temperatures and despite your temp sitting around thirty-seven degrees. Because you are wrapped in bandages, you have no ability to control your body temperature, so Carolyn and I discussed the design of some outfits for you that may suit. I'll see if Joan could make something up. Your mattress from last night will need to be remodelled because you can get your legs right over the wings, which defeats the purpose. This would be mark five.

Carolyn's journal, Day 142, Saturday 8 May 2004
Today, Katrina came and as always is a great help. We had

days of progress

dinner out in the cafe, with Sophie at the table. She really enjoyed the day but it tired her out immensely – we'll see how the night goes. Carolyn has a cross-country pram that she will lend us, which will enable us to go for walks.

Letter to Sophie, Day 143, Sunday 9 May 2004
Mother's Day. We woke you at 10.45 am to have breakfast together. We then took you for a walk – you love the fish. Catherine, John, Kate, Will and Ollie arrived and so did Linda, Wayne and Lillie with McDonald's, so we sat in the cafe for dinner. We are happy that your temperature and stats are stable. Your skin is healing really well and I hope that you are looking good in the bath on Monday. Mitchell has been drawing you beautiful pictures and Lillie did today too. We put you prone at 6.30 tonight; you were so tired, you were asleep in your chair. I hope that you sleep through the night!

It's important that we get you into a nightly routine before you go home, so we have another twenty-one days to break your habit of waking up in the night. I will see if not sleeping in your room will help you settle. Last night, you were awake for an hour, saying 'wake up, Dad!' in the biggest shout you could.

Carolyn's journal, Day 143, Sunday 9 May 2004
Mitchell woke me with Ron at 7.30 am to give me flowers and chocolates. We woke Sophie and went outside for a Mother's Day breakfast. Lots of visitors, so we walked and we talked; we took rides in the lifts and explored various corners of the hospital. Plaster casts on have limited Sophie's playtime, so the walks have been good therapy.

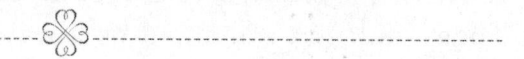

Letter to Sophie, Day 144, Monday 10 May 2004
A wonderful sleep: fourteen hours uninterrupted – a first. A new glove for your right hand was trialled by Nadia [a neoprene mitt that enabled Sophie to grasp paintbrushes, encouraging large arm movements to increase her mobility]. Sandra came with me to talk to the sewing department about clothes for you. Joan, the volunteer who made your beautiful fairy dress, has made you some clothes that are Velcroed together. Your dress is beautiful.

At lunchtime, you got frustrated about not being able to use scissors and started spitting – you do that when you are tired as well. Lisa came with dough, painting, music and puppets and at 4.30 pm we packed up. Your plaster casts went on, then we went for a walk around the hospital and watched videos. At dinner time, you were very happy but kept asking for chicken-noodle soup, chocolate, apple, banana in an attempt to put off going to sleep.

Carolyn's journal, Day 144, Monday 10 May 2004
This morning, Sophie woke up to ask, 'Let's visit fish.' She was due for a dressing change, so we started at 10.30 am. Soph cried in the bath with movements but was great for the dressings – we rubbed sorbolene into her skin and I felt remorse at her broken body again. It is just so sad, her beautiful face full of expectation and wonder and a scarred body – my precious child. After dinner, I left the room so Soph would settle and will return at 10 pm.

Letter to Sophie, Day 145, Tuesday 11 May 2004
Soph, you slept till 8.30 am, when I asked you to get ready for your Wiggles visit. All the Wiggles came and you were so happy. Lilly, Molly and Mitch came too. Mitchell watched,

days of progress

Lilly and Molly played with the Wiggles toys and Molly danced sitting down. You wanted to play your guitar just like Murray and did a very good job strumming and singing. You got a new wheelchair today and came off IV morphine. I left before lunch to have a meeting at home with Mary, so Mitchell had the afternoon at home and I tidied your room and sorted out your wardrobe. I met Eleanor Rose today; she is a beautiful baby girl. Trudy and Zach sent you the biggest hug and kiss and will come and visit so you can meet Eleanor Rose soon.

Letter to Sophie, Day 146, Wednesday 12 May 2004
I arrived back at hospital after a busy time of meetings in the morning. We met Katy, Olivia's mum, at midday so that we could arrange for Amanda and Laura [from the Roundhouse] to visit and to explain what happened the day of the accident. I think it's important for us to know, so that we can help you to have an understanding too. There are a lot of people who want to help and support us, and we will take up their offers as soon as it is appropriate.

You did very well at the dressing change, with no nitrous. You were spitting at Lyn because you were tired and I said that I would tell Sandra. You said, 'Don't tell Sandra,' so I said, 'Say sorry to Lyn,' and you did.

Catherine rings every day to see how you are. You really enjoy your walks in the wheelchair around the hospital. It means you have to try very hard to sit upright yourself, which tires you out. You fell asleep at 6.30 pm and turned prone at 7.30 pm.

You have received so many more gifts and letters and cards; the messages are inspiring, and I hope they will provide you with inspiration in the future. They have certainly helped me on our journey together. It would be lovely to have a book put together for you. You are a bright light each day and I miss you when I'm not with you.

Carolyn's journal, Day 146, Wednesday 12 May 2004
Keith, a firefighter who attended the accident scene, visited again today. Surgery scheduled for Tuesday next week. Yesterday, Ron sorted out a smaller wheelchair that we can use, and Sophie's IV morphine was stopped.

Letter to Sophie, Day 147, Thursday 13 May 2004
Today, we saw the mobile zoo, which Carol arranged. You and Mitchell loved touching the echidna, lizard, snake, croc, cockatoo and frog. This afternoon, you went up to the sensory room in the surgical ward. It's fantastic. We got you rolling and in different positions. Mitchell had fun there too: it has a fish theme and lights and buttons to push.

You started talking about the fire again today, so I spoke to Sandra again about that, and to get help with answering questions from people. We are all going to have to learn this together. I know deep down it's because people are inquisitive and that they care, but a lot of times they don't know how to show it.

Dad went to the plastic-industry charity golf day and said a few words at the dinner afterwards. He is due to speak at the Humpty Dumpty dinner tomorrow night too; they raise funds for North Shore Hospital.

Carolyn's journal, Day 147, Thursday 13 May 2004
A good sleep; awake at 3–4 am. I asked Soph to sing me songs to put me to sleep: 'Baa Baa Black Sheep', 'Rock-a-Bye Baby', 'Twinkle Twinkle', so that she would settle. Today, Soph said, 'Shhhhhhh – that's the noise fire makes. It's hot – whew

days of progress

wheew,' like she was blowing it out. We went outside and there were construction sounds in one of the wards; she said, 'That scares me,' because it was loud. Katy said yesterday that Olivia had startled at loud noises after the accident. I spoke to Sandra, who will attend the meeting with Laura, Amanda and Geata.

Mitchell and Soph had a lovely time in the tactile room in surgical ward, although I'm sensing things are a little tough on Mitchell and he is craving attention. People are stopping to ask what happened to Sophie. I am wary of saying things in front of her and need counselling on how to go about this.

Letter to Sophie, Day 148, Friday 14 May 2004
Mitchell and I arrived in your room at ten. You said to me, 'Mitchell didn't say good morning to me, Mitchell didn't say good morning to me,' and got quite upset. Mitchell had his eyes on the TV set instead. You had a bath in the big bath today, which was great work. You met the bandaged bear and we had sausage sandwiches. Mitchell spent an hour with Sandra and is going for a sleepover with Lilly because Daddy is speaking at the Humpty Dumpty Foundation dinner at Balmoral. Grandma is going, as are Linda and Wayne and Katrina and John; it's his first official speech for a charity dinner.

Your line is playing up, which is a huge shame; we all really hoped it would last till Tuesday. You did really well on the mat in the sensory room, rolling and reaching and throwing a ball. We put weights on your legs for counterbalance, so you would use your abdominal muscles to sit up. I am so proud of you for trying so hard.

Carolyn's journal, Day 148, Friday 14 May 2004
Feel down today. We had a picnic barbecue lunch with Sophie, Grandma Joy and Russell. Mitchell and I spent half an hour

together before it was time for him to see Sandra. I'll be in bed by ten tonight; I was told I looked tired by one of the PICU nurses today.

Letter to Sophie, Day 149, Saturday 15 May 2004
We had a gate-pass today, which allowed us to go with Katrina to Parramatta Park for a picnic. We headed back to the room to have a rest – I sat behind you in bed. Maree and Maria arrived with essential oils to smell. Maria made up a special blend for Mitchell, you and me. We then took a walk to Careflight, and the pilots and doctors came to say hello.

Your dad did really well last night at the Humpty Dumpty dinner and got a standing ovation. They raised funds for the paediatric division at Royal North Shore Hospital, where you were first taken and stabilised – that helped save your life.

Carolyn's journal, Day 149, Saturday 15 May 2004
After a slightly restless sleep, I discussed with Margaret [Maroney] the plan of Ron and I sleeping in another room to see if Sophie settles more easily in the early hours, so that we are not in a position to pander to her multiple requests. Andy looked at her line and got it to flush – it's very positional and had grown *Pseudomonas* on it. Hopefully, it will last till Tuesday. Sophie was very happy this evening and very funny. Mitchell was overtired and struggling for attention.

Letter to Sophie, Day 150, Sunday 16 May 2004
You had an unsettled sleep because you were vomiting so didn't get turned prone. You, Mitchell and I went for a long walk around the oval and collected flowers and stones. Back to the

room for a rest, where you vomited again three times (there is a tummy bug going around). Beth arrived, so we decided to take a walk up to Westmead train station for some trainspotting. You did really well and have not vomited since.

Tomorrow, Geata, Amanda and Laura will be visiting; you are very excited about it. Also seeing Lisa again. We have decided on a lot of games to play with Lisa already, especially up in the sensory room. Mitchell loves it there too, so I promised him we could go there later in the week.

Carolyn's journal, Day 150, Sunday 16 May 2004
Ron had a rough night with Sophie, who vomited continually from 1 am and had diarrhoea. Mitchell sad and agitated about going home and has cried a few times today about it – it breaks my heart to see him sad.

Letter to Sophie, Day 151, Monday 17 May 2004
Geata, Laura and Amanda arrived at 9 am, and we had a good discussion about the accident. You did very well in the bath today, although you cry when Sarah does physio and the bandages come off. We took Lyn for a walk to see the fish with the girls and then went to find Grandma Joy. Trish, your PICU nurse, came by to say farewell before leaving for Africa.

Wendy Parsonage came by; her daughter Penny had an accident in 1969 – seventy-five-per-cent third-degree burns. I saw a photo of her; she looks beautiful and has two happy, healthy children and a wonderful husband.

You had a finger prick today to cross-match your blood; you cry a lot for those. Two Vegemite sandwiches for lunch, then chicken soup and chicken for dinner. You went prone at 8 pm but weren't happy with the pillow. You can try my feather pillow tonight if you wake and we'll see how we go.

Looking forward to more physio exercises tomorrow. You are a star!

Carolyn's journal, Day 151, Monday 17 May 2004
Had a meeting with Geata, Amanda and Laura to gain understanding of the accident. Amanda defied all recommendations to stay out of the building so that she could pull all the children from the room.

A good bath, although I feel sad each time I massage Sophie with sorbolene. Theatre going ahead Thursday afternoon – the last for some time.

Letter to Sophie, Day 152, Tuesday 18 May 2004
A great day, because you sat up for yourself for about fifteen minutes on and off at crèche-playgroup. You had a great time at story- and song-time; you almost clapped your hands. You held a ball with both your hands today. The pain-team doctor came to see you and made sure you got your low-dose ketamine post-op. You had surgery today, a contracture release for your finger and neck. We hope this graft takes, because it means we will be able to head home sooner rather than later. You will need to have further operations this year but at this stage we don't know when. It also depends on how your skin goes and if any breaks down.

You had a happy, busy day and that is how all the doctors and nurses will see you – a happy girl who will rise to each challenge and overcome it with your determination and direct approach. You wiggled around so much last night your head bandage fell off by morning. We tried five pillows and only got you comfy turning you supine. We did get a four-hour block of sleep – hooray!

Letter to Sophie, Day 153, Wednesday 19 May 2004
This morning, we got you into your chair and Lisa spent time with you before your plaster casts went on. I fed you chicken-noodle soup, which went on for an hour and a half; that's the time dinner usually takes. Your favourite saying is 'come here, Mummy', and I have to get really close – right next to your head – and we will have a chat. If I'm not close enough, you say 'no, right here, Mummy'.

Your morphine and ketamine are reduced to half, so we'll see how you go overnight. Your temperatures are still high, although you are on antibiotics. Andy is keen to take your central line out tomorrow to stop any further risk of infection. Today, we met up with the Wood family, and Caroline and I talked about what to expect when we go home and how much help we might need. We have had a number of offers from lots of well-wishers and I think we'll be taking them up on those.

Carolyn's journal, Day 153, Wednesday 19 May 2004
Soph's milestones we are proud of:
– scratching her nose on Monday
– sitting up for a couple of minutes on Tuesday
– sitting in her wheelchair post-op Wednesday for half an hour.

Her injuries still break my heart and I lie awake at night and think what could have been if the car keys had been turned off, if more than one person had helped Amanda, if the fire extinguisher was appropriate. These things I think in the quiet moments when I picture Soph on fire and I feel desperately sad that she had to suffer through that. Despite all the inspiring victories that she has achieved, she is still my baby girl.

Letter to Sophie, Day 154, Thursday 20 May 2004
I woke this morning at 8.30 am and shortly afterwards you woke with the most beautiful smile on your face, saying 'Mummy'; it melted my heart. Dot and Anne, the volunteers, came while I had lunch, made some calls, got some copying organised and made appointments. This afternoon, Connie took off all morphine and antibiotics in anticipation of Dr Andy taking your line out. At around 3 pm, he tried and it didn't come easily, which meant immediate fasting for theatre. I postponed my night at home and Beth took Mitchell to footy. You are on the emergency list; it's 8.30 pm and we are still waiting.

Carolyn's journal, Day 154, Thursday 20 May 2004
You know with Soph that things rarely go to plan, and when they do it is a bonus. Andy in to pull her line but it didn't come, so we are on the emergency list for theatre. And so we wait. I had to put off taking Mitchell to footy because of theatre and I feel that I have let him down again. He is a champion through this too! I feel that I have missed out on six months of caring for Mitchell.

Letter to Sophie, Day 155, Friday 21 May 2004
I left the hospital and arrived home last night at 11.45 pm, after you returned from theatre having had your line removed – hooray. Dad took you for walks around the hospital today to see the birds, gardens and fish. Lyn came at lunchtime and dressed you up with your orange fairy outfit, then put orange nail polish on. Captain Starlight came to visit and sang you songs. We went up to the sensory room together – you, Dad, Mitchell, Sarah, Lisa and I – and you did some physio and played.

    Back in your room, your neck is really sore and you cry a lot to make us aware your 'neck and head hurt'; we put

days of progress

pillows under you on each side. We are not allowed to put a pillow under your head. Because you can't go prone, we are not allowed to have you seated in bed as you are not getting enough hip flexion, so your bed is on a severe tilt to enable you to see the TV. Bedtime is well overdue but your breakthrough morphine has kicked in and you are in a very good mood. If I stayed in the room, you would just want to chat, so I'm taking time out for a cuppa and to write your diary.

Carolyn's journal, Day 155, Friday 21 May 2004
I went home last night after we settled Sophie after theatre. Mitchell ran to my room this morning, saying 'Mummy!' We had lots of cuddles. We had a look at a house today, giving us an idea of what we could find that might be suitable for Sophie long-term. Lunch at home with Mum, then back to hospital. I'm very concerned about Sophie's hand in the splint – it's at such an acute angle, it's shaped like a banana.

Letter to Sophie, Day 156, Saturday 22 May 2004
Catherine, Mandy and Margaret [Henry] came to look after you while I spent time with Kerry Griffin. She was one of the mums who was first on the scene at the accident. She gave me her account of events and, while her recollection differed from Amanda's, the facts remain the same and it helped me to fit some pieces together.

I am often in awe of your acceptance and tolerance for the situation and how your spirit shines through. I believe that you have a special role on this earth and that is to unite people. I am truly blessed to be your mother and you are blessed to have such a caring brother, who whispers in your ear when you are sad, and a dad whose sense of humour will outlast the sad times for you.

Carolyn's journal, Day 156, Saturday 22 May 2004
I brought Sophie in for a visit to Ron and Mitchell [in the Delezios' hospital room] at 9 am. We took her for a walk, then her bath was due at 10.30 – Ron at the helm. I checked on him at 11.30 and he was in tears. The large wounds left where the contractures were released were confronting. Andy said we could have Sophie sleep in our room on the nights of no dressing change if we wanted. I met with Kerry and learnt some more about the accident. It fills me with an incredible sadness. Kerry said she saw Sophie curled in a ball face down as she was pulled out from under the car.

Letter to Sophie, Day 157, Sunday 23 May 2004
Breakfast at the cafe, then we all went to Parramatta Park and you kicked a ball. You are getting the hang of being in the wheelchair, saying 'push, Mummy' and 'stop'. After lunch, you and I went for a really long walk. We fed the ducks and we went to Westmead train station for some trainspotting; we were out for two hours.

We are trying to spend more time out of your room in anticipation of you coming to our hospital bedroom to sleep. We will work through a plan this week of what is needed to come home. We might even be able to go home for a couple of hours! We are fine-tuning your meds, dressing change, physio and feeds to make it a manageable transition but we will be going home soon; if you don't get any infections, it will be within the next three weeks. It's an exciting time – scary, too, but joyous, because it will be the start of our new life together as a family.

Carolyn's journal, Day 157, Sunday 23 May 2004
A cloak that doesn't offer any comfort but becomes oppressive

and heavy: these are the flashback images from the trauma I felt after the accident. I shed the cloak and give it wings to fly away free into the distance.

A happy day. Sophie sparkled. Pam and Susan say the new grafts look large and deep but will fill out in about two weeks.

chapter thirteen
exit strategy

For Sophie and her family, leaving hospital was never going to be as easy as just walking out the door. There is a battery of medications and equipment to be prepared for their return home, for a start. Then there is the accumulation of six months' worth of books, toys, mementoes and clothes to haul home. The teddy bears alone could fill a family-sized car.

Then there is the learning curve: Ron and Carolyn have to learn how to do Sophie's plasters and how to administer her intravenous medication. They also have to find a kindergarten that will embrace Sophie and her unique physical requirements. Looking further ahead, they need to start looking for a school that will be willing to create the kind of physical environment that will allow Sophie to be comfortable and relatively independent.

The Delezios' immediate goal, though, is moving to the Care by Parent ward, where Ron and Carolyn will take charge of Sophie's daily needs.

Letter to Sophie, Day 158, Monday 24 May 2004
The days are getting busier as we plan our exit. You were up and mobile at 7.45 am to walk to Parramatta Park. Back to your room for meds and talking exit strategy with the teams involved. A bath at 10.30 and nitrous used. Finished just before 1 pm, when Grandma Joy joined us for lunch.

Then it was time to trial your prams. You were so excited and said, 'Let's go!' Then, time to have your knees X-rayed. At 3 pm, we met with Nadia to trial a new wheelchair. Joan made you a new dress, which you proudly showed off. Back to the room to have plasters on and a rest.

We went to the restaurant but you became too uncomfortable so we went back to my room to finish dinner. You were asleep on the couch at 7 pm, so I put you prone at 7.30. It's 10.30 and I have had a call from the nurses to say you are upset, so I'll head back to your room to sleep tonight. I love you.

Carolyn's journal, Day 158, Monday 24 May 2004
I don't know why I feel fragile but I do. I've alerted all teams to get ready for phase-out and am being trained in dressings and monitors. Pain management is being fine-tuned, as is physio. I'm starting a list of what we need. I feel sad each night when I go to bed at the moment. At the dressing change, I couldn't look too closely at Sophie's back after seeing her hand. I massage her broken body with cream. I focus on her eyes and feel faint for the second time during a dressing change. Sophie's skin is largely healed but has raw areas still where the skin breaks down. Soph is tired and sad.

Letter to Sophie, Day 159, Tuesday 25 May 2004
Beth came to playgroup with us this morning. You had a sad morning and didn't want to do too much. You were a little sad

overnight, with quite a few tears, although you were easy to settle. We had a little rest in your bed, then went to see Beth off.

At 1.45 pm, you needed to go prone so that physio could mould you a new hip splint. This is so you can wear it overnight if going prone proves to be a problem. Louise and Dave came for the afternoon, which gave me time to meet with Sandra. Dad arrived with Mitchell, which worked out well because Dorothy [the Dinosaur], Captain Feathersword and Anthony from the Wiggles arrived at 5.30 pm and stayed for about half an hour, singing 'Bow Wow' and the Dorothy song.

You ate some spaghetti bolognese for dinner and we trialled Charlotte's pram. I hope the weather is good tomorrow so we can try it outside.

Carolyn's journal, Day 159, Tuesday 25 May 2004
Sophie is really sad and I wonder if it is because of the diazepam withdrawal. She wants me to do things 'now' and, while it is always a balance to manage her needs with her demands, I can't help but feel there is a general frustration within her that must be monitored. I met with Sandra and acknowledged that my true test will be when we get back home in terms of management of stress and how we manage family life in the future.

Letter to Sophie, Day 160, Wednesday 26 May 2004
We had a good night, with you having a huge sleep-in till 10.45 am, the two previous days having been really busy. You did really well at your dressing change, with no nitrous used.

At 12.30 pm, we left you with Catherine and Grandma Joy because Daddy and I met with Carrie and Sandra and Siobhan [Connelly, Burns clinical-nurse consultant] to discuss our planned exit from hospital. There is a lot to arrange but first stop is going up to the Care by Parent ward, which means we will effectively be discharged and we will be responsible for your care. There are two nurses, in case we have problems during the day, but none at night, so Daddy and I will sleep with you during this time and only go home during the day. We have all teams working out timings of phase-out on certain drugs and antibiotics, and arranging plaster casts and additional tests.

You had the opportunity to meet Katherine, a little girl who has prosthetic limbs. You got on really well with her – she lives in Forster. Daddy was impressed with how well she walked and ran. He met her mother, and Sandra came too. Daddy was really proud of you.

Carolyn's journal, Day 160, Wednesday 26 May 2004
Met with Endocrinology team today, who will review Sophie after Betadine baths are stopped (prolonged use of Betadine can lead to thyroid problems). Infectious Diseases doctor said knee X-ray showed rough edges on right leg bone. This could be osteomyelitis. X-ray from Monday shows improvement, so it may not be, but needs to be followed up in a couple of weeks. Pain-management drugs not reduced because of Sophie's sadness yesterday – diazepam will be reduced again tomorrow.

There are so many matters that need to be tidied up before we go home: how to bandage if a full dressing change is ever needed, etc. Therese came over to harmonise. Mum arrived and so did Catherine. I left at 3 pm to come home. Went to skin-cancer clinic to have spots burnt off. Read stories at Mitchell's kindy. Met Fiona [kindy director] for a review of how he is travelling and told her that we will most likely walk Soph to kindy with Mitchell. Takeaway with Mandy and Margaret [Henry] and Augusto [Mandy's flatmate] for Ma's birthday dinner completed a very busy day.

Letter to Sophie, Day 161, Thursday 27 May 2004
Today, I went to watch Mitchell at gym and met Nadia at some land we are looking at. We then went to Balgowlah North Public School and met the principal. I left Nadia having discussions with him with respect to 'Sophie's special needs'. They already have special-needs children and the layout of the school is well suited for wheelchair access.

Mitchell and I then dropped Grandma at the airport; we sent her off to Canberra for a long weekend. Mitchell and I dropped something off at the factory for Dad and then headed back to hospital.

Melissa arrived just as we did, so you got to play with Michael, Jessica and Christopher for two hours. Then Mitchell lay next to you in bed while you watched a bit of TV together. You both had pasta for dinner. Daddy and I have been administering your drugs and feeds. It's a very exciting, full-on time!

Carolyn's journal, Day 161, Thursday 27 May 2004
After the skin-cancer clinic yesterday, I went to the baby shop we always bought from and got a bit teary when asking for bed brackets so Sophie doesn't tumble out of bed. I have said to Sandra I think the hardest time will be me going home.

In the morning, I had my first leg wax in eight months – hooray! It felt liberating. Una, a lady from Maree's healing circle, offered me a healing treatment for nothing and I said to her that I am just surrendering to everyone and saying yes, because we need all the help we can get.

Letter to Sophie, Day 162, Friday 28 May 2004
We were up and out in the cross-country pram at 9.30 am for a walk to the post office at the main hospital. Back for your bath after picking up a new outfit from the volunteers' shop –

Joan made you some trousers and a hat. We went mid-dressing change to have an echo scan on your heart. Your liver, bladder and kidneys were given an ultrasound.

Back to your room for meds, and Mitchell and Dad arrived. I took you for a walk to the chemist to have balloons blown up and the chemist gave you a doctor doll that has zips, buttons, laces and Velcro. We visited the library, to return some books, and also the chapel. Dad took over, showing you and Mitchell our new bedroom in the Care by Parent section on level two. Mitchell had a good time with Sandra and she wants to see you soon too.

Lee and Mark came to visit and told us stories about their great four-wheel-drive expedition to Kakadu and Katherine Gorge. Crocodiles everywhere and some even that fought each other – they are very territorial. You fall fast asleep after another busy day. We love you.

Carolyn's journal, Day 162, Friday 28 May 2004
I learnt how to do meds today. We finished Sophie's dressings in her bedroom; Mitchell saw Sophie's trunk exposed for the first time but seemed unfazed by it. Ron took the children off to visit our new room. Soph seemed very accepting, as we had already been up to the room. Soph asleep by 8 pm in her new outfit and matching hat from Joan.

Letter to Sophie, Day 163, Saturday 29 May 2004
Daddy and Mitchell and you and I had breakfast in our room. You arrived at 9 am with croissants. We then met Catherine, John, Kate, Will and Ollie in the cafe, and Katrina and John arrived. They were here to help move shelves into the family room at home, which is your new play space. Dad and Mitchell went home with them late in the afternoon because Mitchell had a birthday party in the morning.

We had another look at your new bedroom. It's exciting and scary at the same time. Janice and Russell came to visit in the afternoon as well. We gave Aaron a music voucher as a thank you for sharing his story with us. We went for a walk this afternoon to the park and to the train station. You were so tired that you were asleep at 5.15 pm.

You woke quite a few times in the early hours, asking for water or change of nappy. Sometimes, it's hard to ignore your requests, despite them being a habit. We walk the hospital corridors and visit the various artworks and sculptures: the bandaged bear climbing the pole in the atrium, the wrought-iron bed and the girl covered in hearts who says, 'I who have nothing bring love so you can grow in a world of hope.'

Carolyn's journal, Day 163, Saturday 29 May 2004
Mitch and I slept together and woke to a knock at the door; it was 9 am! And Sophie knocked. We went out for a quick walk in the park at 4.30 pm and to visit the trains. We are administering the meds ourselves; diazepam is being dropped first, then clonidine.

Letter to Sophie, Day 164, Sunday 30 May 2004
We are up and out by 9.30 am, ready for our walk in the baby jogger. We walk around Parramatta Park and to Westmead station to see the trains. Back for meds and a bite of lunch. I get fed by a lovely Greek family whose daughter Sarah – in a pink wheelchair – is back in for a couple of weeks. Mitchell and Daddy arrive back after the party and we go for another walk around the oval.

The helipad is in front of Westmead Hospital. On our earlier walk, we saw the helicopter take off; you said you didn't like it, it was too noisy. Janet and David [Binks] arrived, as did Catherine and Antoni and Jeff from the Wiggles, who spent close to an hour with us just chatting. You loved to show him your Jeff dolls and the songs they sing. When everyone left, it was time to head back for dinner but you were asleep by 6 pm. We are leaving your NG tube out to see how you do. We shall review tomorrow – you have no tubes!

Carolyn's journal, Day 164, Sunday 30 May 2004
Soph slept well, except for the usual calls for water. Two vomits, two poos and an NG tube vomited out. I'm unsure what we should do about that if we are in Care by Parent. It worries me and I feel sad about the transition, although I know it must be made. I feel teary on return to the ward. I understand they will come up to us in Care by Parent if we need it. Thank goodness – I feel uncertain and anxious about a move home. I let Sophie look at herself in the mirror today. After a while, she said, 'My ear's gone.' I said the ear was still there, just the skin around the edge wasn't.

Letter to Sophie, Day 165, Monday 31 May 2004
You managed your bath well and were measured for your first Jobst garments (special pressure garments to help your skin grafts heal well). This will help shorten the time dressing changes take.

We had another look at your new room and we took some of your things upstairs. Rather than being rushed, we have decided to move up tomorrow, once we have arranged all pumps, drugs, etc. I thank God and Mary MacKillop for the second chance we have of 'life with Sophie'. It is sad to be leaving Clubbe Ward and the familiarity of nursing staff and your lovely room but it is progress, and it's exciting to be moving upstairs to our new life together as a family.

There is a lot of stuff to tidy up from your room and

wonderful treasures that so many well-wishers have sent you. I feel strongly they are a part of you and shall remain close to your bed. We go for walks around the hospital and so many people want to stop and chat to you and see how you're doing, because they all care very much about you. I think, though, you get a bit sick of the interruptions, because your standard line now is 'Let's go, Mummy'.

Carolyn's journal, Day 165, Monday 31 May 2004
Sophie is awake and cries in the early hours of the morning – she achieves quite a volume! Got organised for the morning with planning meetings for our departure. We met with Andy to have an overview of Sophie's future care and started taking things to a new room. Sophie is very excited. We have a few things to arrange – equipment/meds, etc. for a transfer on Tuesday. I packed up this evening after rocking Soph to sleep. I hold her close and feel immense sadness. I wept tonight for our future and for our past, but it's time to move on to the next phase in our life with Sophie. I pray to God to help me through. I feel all the grief well up inside me again at this time.

Letter to Sophie, Day 166, Tuesday 1 June 2004
Today is moving day – we move from Clubbe Ward to Care by Parent room number six. It's a busy day, having your new hats [pressure dressings] fitted and then off to playgroup.

We went back to the new room and settled in some more, although your bed didn't arrive till mid-afternoon. Keryn, one of the volunteers, helped us move while Grandma Joy spent time wheeling you around the hospital. You love to go to the Starlight Room and visit Captain Starlight, who sings you songs and makes funny faces at you. I met with Debra from PR, who was arranging a press conference for Thursday with the premier and state minister for Health. I signed the official discharge forms and when Dad arrived we had a nice dinner in the room.

You were fast asleep when Dad carried you down to Clubbe Ward for your 8 pm meds (these can't be kept in the Care by Parent ward). You stayed asleep the whole time. It was lovely having Dad in the room, although I don't think he slept too well in the bed – he kept complaining about how lumpy it was. We left some of your decorations in the playroom at Clubbe Ward: stars, Dorothy, rainbows, sea horses and turtles. We will leave the weather painting for the ward too. You did say, 'I want go sleep my other room,' at bedtime but soon were happy to stay here.

Carolyn's journal, Day 166, Tuesday 1 June 2004

Today was moving day and it was busy with any number of meetings. We met staff from the minister's office in between finding syringes, water, etc. to give Sophie meds at the appropriate time. It was great having a meal with Ron and weeping together for what has been lost and talking through what has been gained.

Letter to Sophie, Day 167, Wednesday 2 June 2004

Your new suit was fitted today after your bath. You were so proud of it that you didn't want to wear your dress, so we walked around the hospital in your purple 'zoot suit' and nappy. But when you do a poo it's so messy that it means the whole suit has to come off and be washed. Catherine had to borrow the hairdryer from Clubbe Ward and it took the two of us an hour and a quarter to change you.

Daddy and Grandma had been at a lunch for the sponsors of the Humpty Dumpty Foundation, where Daddy was presented with a trip to Bali for six days for four people. That would be a fun trip to do; we have always wanted to go to Bali.

We tidied your bedroom because we have been told part of the leading-edge technology used on your back graft is going to be announced in a press conference tomorrow. We now understand why the premier as well as the health minister wanted to meet you. In the meantime, the volunteers have again helped out. Anne is particularly lovely and wheeled you around looking for the pain-team doctor to say goodbye and give her a picture – she's been on your pain team and has done a great job.

Carolyn's journal, Day 167, Wednesday 2 June 2004
A busy start to the day, with Ron heading off to receive our Bali trip officially. Mum joined him. Sophie and I did the rounds of bath time, being fitted for new suits, physio, weekly meeting, meds, meeting people who wanted to say hello to Sophie and pass on best wishes.

Letter to Sophie, Day 168, Thursday 3 June 2004
The day was always destined to be a busy one. Up at 8 am for meds at Clubbe. Daddy and I had to shower and have you at physio by 9 am; you did another big poo, so it was a very hurried leg dressing before plaster casts came off. Then to the room for the premier to read you some stories, which he did very well – you particularly liked *The Rainbow Fish* [by Marcus Pfister]. The press conference went reasonably well; Dr Peter Maitz and Dr Peter Hayward both spoke very well and it made the news on all the stations. They took footage of you and you were smiling beautifully.

You are starting to tell me you want to go to the toilet, which is great, so we attempted it at a couple of toilets before changing your nappy at the Burns ward. We met with the registrar, who

exit strategy

215

is reviewing your pain chart in terms of vitamins and arranging all the follow-up appointments for your ongoing care. We met with Connie, who is going to make you some trousers and a special seat for the toilet. I went home to see about your team and arrange a few things, which helped me feel better about bringing you home. We hope to do some home visits next week to reorientate you to the home environment. I'm not sure where we will house all your soft toys: there are six big bags and a bed full of them.

Carolyn's journal, Day 168, Thursday 3 June 2004
A press release today meant a meeting with the New South Wales health minister's office and the premier, Bob Carr. Before that, he wanted to read to Sophie. The press conference itself was a shambles, in my opinion, with the minister taking questions about Lebanon in the middle of it – politics! The press coverage on the news was better, though, and I felt a bit more comfortable after seeing it. Physio and various appointments and meetings fill Sophie's day; each day is a step closer to the door, but I have to feel comfortable with everything before I take a step *out* of the door.

Letter to Sophie, Day 169, Friday 4 June 2004
A great day. You achieved two huge milestones. Firstly, you asked to go to the toilet and did poos and wees on your own. I supported you. I was so proud; we told everyone we knew. The other milestone was going in the car seat in the car to go shopping at Bonds. That was with Catherine, Mitchell, Daddy and me – we went to get new T-shirts.

You did good physio today and even said when you were lying down, 'Mummy, my arm not hurt me.' You have progressed in that you have two plaster casts on each wrist but splints on each elbow instead of casts. We are fine-tuning a special bench for you to lean on so you can draw. It's a bit like an upside-down highchair. You did well in your bath again and now have a pink suit, which looks really smart. Tonight, I had to put you prone: we tie your legs together and wrap your hips in a sheet so your bottom is not lifting.

Carolyn's journal, Day 169, Friday 4 June 2004
A dressing change/bath this morning and a new suit lined with plastic around the buttocks so that poo doesn't cover Sophie like last time. We met some people who had wanted to give Sophie a quilt, then some other people whose son had been burnt seventy-five per cent two years ago.

Sophie's night-time regime is tough: tied legs, tied hips, two elbow splints, wrists in plaster and a pillow that is not comfortable. She cried for ages. It's so distressing but needs to be done to help her right leg stop from lifting due to contracture and muscle tension. It is an impossible situation and difficult to deal with, as Sophie is in such discomfort. It is more than any child should have to endure and it puts Ron and me under immense stress working out how to deal with it.

Letter to Sophie, Day 170, Saturday 5 June 2004
A beautiful day today. We had a lazy start after you woke lots in discomfort: arms, legs, neck, back. You were on your back, prone, then with the pillow on one side and then the other. We had a picnic outside with John and Kate, Will, Ollie, Katrina, which was lovely. Katrina has been wonderful, spending Saturdays with us and entertaining both you and Mitchell. We got you rolling on the mat and Mitchell loves to show you his gym exercises – you love to see him do them too.

We are slowly packing up the unit downstairs in an effort to get things home but not arrive with huge numbers of bags to unpack. I think we will be home within two weeks and I look forward to the challenge. It's also a little scary, as we want to do the absolute best for you. We tried you in your other car seat today to check which one will give you the most support; you seem to be most comfortable in your old one, so we'll keep that in the car for now. We are planning a trip home tomorrow to see how you go with reorientation at home. It will be great!

Carolyn's journal, Day 170, Saturday 5 June 2004
I will be forever grateful for Katrina's weekly support; it has eased the burden immensely because, as Sophie has been getting better, she has also been getting more demanding and frustrated at her lack of ability to do things that Mitchell does and keep up with Mitchell. I feel very torn between Sophie's demands and Mitchell's demands and will have to be very firm with them both about what I can cope with. We are getting close to the end of our hospital stay and will definitely be out of here in two weeks. I will not go home without some home help in place. I feel that this tests Ron and me hugely at times, and it will be those issues we will have to work through if we can. Sophie must have woken about eight times last night and I'm so tired.

chapter fourteen
'we're lucky'

Before Sophie's big move home, the family do some 'trial runs', visiting first for the day, then sleeping over. The gradual adjustment is necessary – for Sophie, to ease the shock after many months in hospital, and, for her family, to feel comfortable with the responsibility that will now be theirs. Their delight with being together again is mingled with anxious anticipation – and a little sorrow at leaving the tight framework of support that the Children's Hospital at Westmead has offered them for half a year.

A short drive from the Delezios' home lies Arranounbai School. Tucked away in bushland behind Sydney's Northern Beaches, Arranounbai brings together children with special needs and those without. Here, Sophie could join a preschool class and have the benefit of the skills and services provided by the Physical Ability Unit (PAU). Located in rooms at Arranounbai, the PAU team includes physiotherapists, occupational therapists and a registered nurse.

Letter to Sophie, Day 171, Sunday 6 June 2004
A celebratory day, with us all going home for a trial run. You were very excited to see your room and toys and swings and pool. I realised we will have to get you a special seat that will keep you safe and give you a variation on your wheelchair. It's going to be a busy time but we all really enjoyed being together again. Grandma Joy came home to a lovely surprise, although we didn't stay too long after she arrived. When we got back to the hospital, Daddy said, 'It's good to be together.' I said, 'We're family,' and you said, 'We're lucky,' and we really really are. We have travelled a long road and are about to start a new journey.

Carolyn's journal, Day 171, Sunday 6 June 2004
A groundbreaking day. We all got our act together by midday and headed home. It was actually to check which car seat was best but we ended up in Seaforth, with Sophie sleeping both ways.

Me returning all my phone messages and the realisation of how damn hard it will be going home. Sophie wants to go here and then there and then here and then there and her only mode of transport today was me. Once home, she doesn't want to sit in her pram. It's exhausting carrying her around all day and frightening climbing down the stairs with her. We arrived at 1 pm and by 4 pm she wanted to go back to hospital.

Letter to Sophie, Day 172, Monday 7 June 2004
We are making progress towards departure, although at times it seems slow. Sophie, you made really good progress with kneeling on a special chair today. The nurses have just about finished your Sophie book [filled with stories from hospital staff] so will do the rounds of Captain Starlight and the volunteers and doctors, physios and play therapists.

You have been asking to go to the toilet very well today and I'm proud of you for doing so. I have extended our option to stay beyond the weekend and will start packing up the unit next week. You did well in your bath today; you love the massage and cream. I'm looking forward to establishing our routine at home and can't wait for you to regain the independence you deserve. You make progress every day and you surprise me with what you achieve.

Carolyn's journal, Day 172, Monday 7 June 2004
Beth and Mum came and helped out with Sophie, and we did domestic stuff and went for a walk. I met with the dietician, and Lisa came by. Bath time is getting easier – we just need to get into a routine of putting cream on Sophie. I am finalising all the things we need to do for Sophie with doctors, etc., which should be finished by the end of this week. I feel in a state of limbo but know this is the right pace for our departure. Sophie is heavy and wants to be carried a lot of the time. I can see trips to the chiropractor will be needed soon.

Letter to Sophie, Day 173, Tuesday 8 June 2004
We left hospital early this morning to arrive at Balgowlah North School, where we met the principal and area rep about Mitchell's and your enrolment. We were very happy with the outcome. There will need to be some modifications, which will start mid next year. We then went home and Mary was waiting for us. Mum cooked a lovely lunch and we all sat up at the table together, which was great. You sat with Mum and Louise watching swimming on TV and fell asleep on the couch. We are going to need a lot of equipment for you, with mats, dressing-change tables and tables and chairs for you to use for play activities. It's just as well we have a storeroom.

Carolyn's journal, Day 173, Tuesday 8 June 2004

A wonderful trip home but I can't help but feel exhausted when I get there. Ron suggests it may be the responsibility of the running of the house when I'm there. I have not had to deal with any of that for six months.

The meeting with the school went well today and I'm happy to go there with both Mitchell and Sophie. We met Jo, Nadia and Siobhan [play therapist] with Julie from NRMA [Insurance] and then Rod at the house to discuss equipment requirements and the practicality of where dressing changes should be done.

Sophie really enjoyed the day. We had Mary and Mum and Louise there to help look after Sophie so we could talk uninterrupted. Sophie can be very demanding, because she wants to be busy and there are limits to where she can sit. It will be a challenge but it is wonderful to be taking the next step together.

Letter to Sophie, Day 174, Wednesday 9 June 2004

We didn't have the best night last night and, as a result, you were really tired all day. We were lucky to have you bathed early, which meant we could catch up with Molly and Lilly. We met a child from a Christian school who had arranged some fund-raising and wanted to present you with the cheque. I met with the dietician about what to expect in relation to your feed regime and what food to supplement it with. Lyn came to physio, as did Grandma Joy, then Lisa and Lyn looked after you while we met with the insurance company. When you are tired, it means you just don't want to do anything and your pain threshold is really low, so you don't tolerate your plaster casts being put on very well. It's a tough day for all concerned.

Carolyn's journal, Day 174, Wednesday 9 June 2004

I feel a haunting sadness for a family of four – the mother, now in North Shore Hospital, has lost her three children in a house fire. The eldest boy, seven, died here last night and it is a stark reminder of how far we have come. I really feel for the mother and her family members, having had to turn off the life support.

We had a shocking night last night, which means a shocking day today in terms of Sophie's ability to cope, interact, do physio, etc. She was uncooperative, temperamental and exhausting, as well as being exhausted. It was her typical non-compliant day. Hopefully, she will have a reasonable night. The principal problem is comfort while sleeping with all the splints in position. We had a team meeting involving the insurance company's rep, who is physio trained and presents to the claim department. We shall see what the response is to our requests next week in anticipation of going home.

Letter to Sophie, Day 175, Thursday 10 June 2004
We had a lovely day today, with a visit from Sally Anne, a parent at your old kindy, and her daughter Lilly Fay. It was beautiful when you were at the aviary: Lilly and you held hands while you watched the birds. Sally Anne brought dress-ups – we played shops and stickers and you did cooking, making apricot balls, which you then gave to physio, Lisa and the nurses at Clubbe Ward. You had a good play session with Lisa, and plaster casts went on.

You didn't eat anything today and have vomited three times tonight. Joan has made you a skirt and top, which look lovely on you. We met a little girl, Katie Tara, and her mother Karen and sister Corey today. Katie Tara has 'lucky legs' [Sophie's name for her prosthetic legs] too but scoots around on her knees at a rate of knots. She ran down the hall with her three-year-old sister and it was delightful. We also met a little boy from Coffs Harbour, Keily, who doesn't have arms. Captain Starlight sang you and Lilly some songs and the clown doctors played some magic tricks with you.

When you vomited this evening, I thought that if this was at home I would be very worried. Karen said she would often just bring Katie Tara straight to Emergency instead of going to the doctor.

Carolyn's journal, Day 175, Thursday 10 June 2004
We met Karen, Katie Tara and Corey today – Peter Hayward had asked them to call by. Katie Tara had meningococcal disease at ten months and lost both her legs. She speeds down the hall with her little sister – she moves amazingly well on her knees. She has prosthetic legs and wears them about half the year.

Soph had a good session with Lisa and then casts went on and we visited Clubbe Ward to say hi to the nurses. Anne, one of the volunteers, offered to babysit while we went out to dinner for Ron's birthday. We went to the cafe so we could have a wine. We have met remarkable people here; it's a real community of people with the most amazing spirits. I feel our lives are enriched because of it. This evening, I have listened to my daughter cry and vomit in pain as she lies prone – her arms in casts and splints, her legs tied.

Letter to Sophie, Day 176, Friday 11 June 2004
I felt like I accomplished something today with arranging all the appliances to go home: pumps, poles and so on. We'll head home for a trial run this weekend and see what we need. We went to physio with Melissa, Michael, Jessica and Christopher, who played with balls while you were in your chair kneeling and being distracted by Lisa. You managed twenty minutes, which was fantastic. You now have your plaster casts on for

three days, so I hope you don't vomit. You crash at 7 pm and we put you prone at 8.30 – we will have to be very strict about your routine because you need to have a decent sleep to be happy and engaging the next day.

Carolyn's journal, Day 176, Friday 11 June 2004
Sophie had a shocking night, with lots of vomits, and pooed in her nappy. She told me at 9 am she was tired, and so was I. Soph only got three hours prone and I was so pleased she was having a bath as there was vomit and poo all over her suit. We will do a stool sample and see if she needs more gas tonight.

She had a good meeting with the pain team and we arranged to collect the evening meds from the ward, rather than Ron waking her. I met with Neville from finance and arranged feeds, pumps, meds, etc. Neville went to pharmacy and appliance centre [for hiring and buying medical equipment and supplies] and dieticians to advise them on our payment process. We don't really fit into the 'norm'.

Letter to Sophie, Day 177, Saturday 12 June 2004
I slept with Mitchell last night and had a good nine hours, which was fantastic. Daddy rang, needing help to clean you after a poo and to get your morning meds from Clubbe Ward. Once we got ourselves organised, we decided to take a trip home to get your bedroom organised, and that's exactly what we did. You sat in your pink chair, and Mitchell and I unpacked. Well, Mitchell and you kept playing with everything as you explored all your toys again – you had such fun. Then you wanted to watch the Wiggles, so I sat you on the Pooh Bear couch. You seemed really happy to be home and very content. You love sitting on the seat swing and swinging high without me holding you.

Carolyn's journal, Day 177, Saturday 12 June 2004
Today, we arranged to go home for the afternoon to get started on the bedroom move. We have a huge amount to move from Sophie's room. We left for hospital about 6.30 pm and Sophie was asleep within ten minutes of being in the car. She managed the day very well.

Letter to Sophie, Day 178, Sunday 13 June 2004
We were up, showered and tidied, ready to go at 9.30 am. We went down to the room with Daddy and Mitchell and packed a few more things for the trip home. There is not much space in the boot with your wheelchair or pram in there. After we got home, John and Kate arrived, and we moved the bedrooms around again. I had you sitting in your pink chair while I unpacked and again you and Mitchell had a lovely time playing with all your toys. We put you to bed at 7 pm and I turned you back from being prone at 8.30 pm. I sat with you for half an hour but you have remained asleep. You seemed happy to settle into your new room.

Carolyn's journal, Day 178, Sunday 13 June 2004
We did Sophie's meds and packed up as much as we could fit in the car. We arrived just before lunch, so we did a hurried tidy up before lunch. Wayne and Lillie came over; so did Louise and Dave and Carolyn and James, Lee and Mark, Katrina and John, Maree and Mary, Catherine and Antoni. Mum finished golf and joined in. Everyone organised the food; Ron cooked a great steak. Caroline, Scott, Lilly and Molly came over as well. We opened a jeroboam of champagne – we thought it was appropriate to celebrate Sophie's homecoming and Ron's birthday. I won it before Mitchell was conceived, so it was a good vintage! Everyone helped with Sophie and kept telling me to watch my back.

I've got the most fantastic friends who just get organised and do. Thank goodness: I felt disorientated and sad and joyous to be home. I have to remember to care for Mitchell in all of this, as I haven't had to be his full-time carer for six months and keep forgetting his mealtime and bath/bedtime routine. I've decided just to take all the help that is offered and see what happens!

Letter to Sophie, Day 179, Monday 14 June 2004
We had a lovely morning. [Friends] Karen Tayla and Brayden took Mitchell to the zoo, and we finished tidying up after the party and arranging your room. It is still nowhere near finished and there are bags of stuff in the back of the garage. I'm not sure what we will do with all your soft toys, Sophie. We headed back to hospital with Mitchell just after lunch and you had a bath, which went well with no pre-med.

Mitchell and I tidied up our unit and got some things ready to go home tomorrow. Katrina and John, Lee and Mark have offered to carry stuff for us. We came upstairs afterwards and you showed the nurses how you can wheel your wheelchair; we were all thrilled. It was a late night by the time we went to bed. You did really well last night, considering it was your first night at home. Somehow, we all rested easier being in adjoining rooms instead of all together.

Carolyn's journal, Day 179, Monday 14 June 2004
Sophie did quite well overnight. Six wakes: four I covered; two Ron did at her request. It is easier to leave her crying when she is in her own room. We will have to sort out mattresses so she is comfortable enough to go prone. Soph seemed very content being at home and I felt the freedom of not being confined to one room!

There is still a lot to arrange and the collection of stuff we have acquired over six months has to be sorted out and put away. We will have to clear out old toys and bring them to the hospital. A bear room open to the public at Bear Cottage [the hospice of the Children's Hospital at Westmead] would be great.

Back for a bath after lunch; Sophie has an infection in her scalp. Cream will need to be used twice a day, which will force us into the twice-daily massage with the cream. Mitchell and I packed up some stuff from the unit ready to take home on Friday. Sophie permitting, it will be an exciting day.

I'm looking forward to some home-cooked meals. I keep thinking Sophie was too beautiful for this world and somehow this is her test – her challenge and ours. All I can think about is that it has got to be for the greater good.

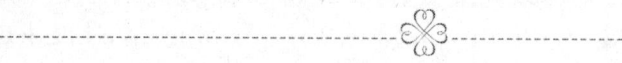

Letter to Sophie, Day 180, Tuesday 15 June 2004
Another busy day, with physio and changing your hat. Every second day, we have to bathe you in special oil and you are on antibiotics four times a day. Today, you helped to feed the fish, as well as meeting the policeman from Parramatta. You were given two Maisy books from the police volunteer, then we went to the library and borrowed more Maisy books. John came to help us move everything from the unit and he took it home and unpacked it into the garage. Mary will come on Thursday to help move some more things and then we can move more again on the weekend.

Carolyn's journal, Day 180, Tuesday 15 June 2004
Sophie wakes on average six times a night, but she is generally easy to get back to sleep. I'm realising just how busy going home will be. Cheri wants to have us doing daily baths and for us to learn how to do plaster casts. Things are progressing with getting us home: Ron met Arranounbai School and Noakes

nursing agency (who will provide home care) and has arranged some quotes to be forwarded to Nadine at NRMA [who has taken over the claim from Julie].

Letter to Sophie, Day 181, Wednesday 16 June 2004
A bath at 9.15 am finished at 11.30 am, then we had physio and Dr Andy did a full review. We went to pathology; you don't like the finger prick and immediately close your hand into a fist. You slept from 2.30 until 6 pm. Lyn came and looked after you and you even slept through your plaster casts going on. You were really pleased to see Daddy arrive back after meetings. I spoke with Lyn to see if she could remain our ward granny, as we will be coming in to have baths on Mondays, Wednesdays and Fridays. We will have meetings after each one and she will be able to take you for walks while we have these. There will be appliance centre, physio, pharmacy requirements as well, so it will be a real help. We will have Mitchell with us on Fridays, so meetings with Sandra will be arranged. We anticipate Sophie working with Sandra over the next few months as well. It is an exciting and daunting time ahead. People say we have a marathon ahead of us but you've been running marathons 24/7 for six months. We had lots of cuddles today, which I really loved.

Carolyn's journal, Day 181, Wednesday 16 June 2004
We got an early start to the day but it was really busy. I met the pain team, who reviewed weaning Sophie off her medications, and we will have a script for diazepam if needed for Sophie to sleep if the splinting regime is increased.

The school Ron met with yesterday has physio and kindy and is prepared to offer Sophie a place immediately; we think this will work well, complemented with a play therapist/day carer and a nurse who can be trained with us.

We may leave Friday or Monday; we will be home over the weekend, though, which will give us another opportunity to arrange things. We are waiting to confirm when Peter Hayward can do a review of Sophie. I still feel incredibly sad when I see Sophie after her dressing change, particularly when there is the green or cream of a breakdown – Sophie has quite a few at present on legs, arm, neck and head.

Letter to Sophie, Day 182, Thursday 17 June 2004
We had lots of meetings to finalise your care arrangements for home. We spend a lot of time having plaster casts put on. The weight of your plaster cast on your left wrist meant it didn't give you the stretch you need, so a new splint will have to be made. You did not have a good night's sleep with Dad last night.

Carolyn's journal, Day 182, Thursday 17 June 2004
An immensely stressful day, with me losing it at Ron at the end for not being back in our room to help with Sophie's head-dressing change before she went to sleep for the night. Her care will have to be timetabled and it will take discipline to stick to, but we need it in order to achieve all in the day we are hoping to achieve.

We did make progress today: appointing a care manager, organising drugs for home and meeting with the pain team. Ron was busy arranging nursing-agency quotes for approval from NRMA. Mary was supposed to be here to help with the move but instead spent time looking after Mitchell while we attended separate meetings till 4 pm. Then it was physio till 5 pm. They are really full days and we still haven't packed up either room completely. I rang Beth and asked if she could come in to help out Friday mornings. It's hard enough achieving all that's necessary in a day with Sophie without having the responsibility of Mitchell.

Letter to Sophie, Day 183, Friday 18 June 2004
Beth arrived to look after you and Mitchell while we went to a meeting, and she packed up some of your toys to go home. You had a really unsettled evening from 7 pm until 10.30: you vomited, pooed, weed and cried a lot. I hope you sleep okay for the rest of the night, as you need a good sleep; it makes your days so much better and we all cope better as a result. You are really excited about going home, which is wonderful.

Carolyn's journal, Day 183, Friday 18 June 2004
An early bath, which Sophie managed well. Beth helped look after Sophie and kept Mitchell entertained while I got a few supplies and ran messages. Sophie slept till 2 pm, when it was sensory-room time, then straight to physio for plaster casts and a new splint. Back to the room for 4 pm to meet the nursing agency.

Catherine came around with Antoni, and we managed to get Sophie's head dressed and legs creamed by seven. Sophie then wet and pooed her nappy; we tried to turn her prone and put splints on but she got so upset she vomited. Her NG tube nearly came out and everyone was really stressed. Her prone mattress had to get washed, her bed changed, her NG pushed back in. Sophie woke at 10.15 pm after a nightmare and was inconsolable. We had to go to Clubbe Ward for breakthrough morphine.

Letter to Sophie, Day 184, Saturday 19 June 2004
We had a leisurely start because you had a shocking night, with dreams, vomits, poos and unsettled behaviour. We were on the road home for the night with a full car again before lunch. You were really demanding all afternoon, just wanting to sit on my knee all the time; it was really tiring and I had a very sore back by the end of the day. We are arranging your room, though,

and have an area designated for all of your medications and dressings, so it's easy to find everything.

You are really happy to be home and there is a noticeable difference in your behaviour. You are more confident and thoroughly enjoy finding all the toys that you had at hospital. It is a hard transition for me to be home; I keep having to remind myself about afternoon teas and dinner for you and Mitchell. It's wonderful having Grandma Joy around to do all that. I really notice the difference in having space – it's wonderful just going into another room.

Carolyn's journal, Day 184, Saturday 19 June 2004
We head home. It always seems such a mad rush – the car is packed with three-quarters of Sophie's stuff just for one night. It is getting really exciting as we get closer to Monday. It is also really tiring. Sophie just wants to sit on my knee; we will have to find a happy balance. If only we had some safe seating. Nadia is arranging some options for us and we might just invest in a foldaway pram. I think Sophie will adapt and, as she gets frustrated with lying or sitting still, she will undoubtedly find a way.

There is an amazing amount of stuff we need to arrange for Sophie but my priority is getting her room functional. We will have a set of drawers as dressing drawers and the workstation may yet function as a change table. I'm tired and stressed and find myself snapping all the time at Mitchell and Ron and Mum, as Sophie screams for attention. I'm looking forward to nursing care to give us some relief from the intensity of her care.

Letter to Sophie, Day 185, Sunday 20 June 2004
You and Mitchell played really well today. I sat you on Mitchell's

bed with the beanbag behind you and used your hands to help shift your weight – the start of your mobility. We got your room a bit more organised and Mitchell's room tidied, then back to hospital overnight for our day of departure. We drove back in the four-wheel drive so we could load it full of stuff, which we did, and Grandma Joy took it home.

Scott has offered to drive us home in a Tarago. I think we'll need it, as there is still lots of stuff to go: equipment, medical supplies. You went to bed at the appropriate time, around 7 pm. I turned you from being prone after two and a half hours. You were crying but even then your manners are beautiful. You cry and say, 'Excuse me, Mummy.' Then, when I've wiped your tears, you say, 'Thank you, Mummy.'

I'm so proud of you – your courage and frankness and the effort you have put in through the past one hundred and ninety days. I hope now we can really work on the rehab phase of your care and that you enjoy doing it. We will be back every second day, so we will continue to see all our hospital friends. They have become our extended family for the last six months. No regrets, though, as now it's time to take the trip home.

Carolyn's journal, Day 185, Sunday 20 June 2004
A busy day finishing Sophie's room and tidying Mitchell's. We only managed to get one bag of toys out to give to the hospital. I will work on this more; his room looks a lot better and now there is less risk of Grandma tripping over things. Sophie will have to learn I can't pick her up all the time. All the same, it was great to be home. One night to go!

chapter fifteen
going home

Home again, and Carolyn revels in the sheer pleasure of being able to move from room to room after the confines of hospital rooms and wards. Carolyn's letter to Sophie is complete for now – from here on, the journal is purely her personal account. Carolyn stops counting the days at Day 203, and the entries become less regular, recording isolated hurdles and milestones as the family moves out of crisis mode at last.

In these private pages, Carolyn vents the frustrations of some days and ponders over the emotional toll this new life and her new job as Sophie's carer is taking on her and her family. The trip to Bali donated to the Delezios by the Humpty Dumpty Foundation is finally possible for them, but Sophie can't go because of the heat and the risk of infection. So she and Carolyn stay at home.

Carolyn's journal, Day 186, Monday 21 June 2004
Hooray! We are all so happy to be home. It was thrilling arriving and knowing that we were here with Sophie and here to

stay. It was exciting leaving hospital: we had a guard of honour with clapping and cheering and a few tears as we left. Thank goodness Scott arranged the Tarago: we still had a heap of stuff to come home.

Sophie arrived and said, 'Let's get into bed – come on, Mummy.' She was so happy. Nursing care arrived at three and it has been a huge relief. It took an hour and a half to change Sophie's head and put cream on her body. This needs to be done twice daily.

Catherine, John, Kate and Will, Beth and Carol Cooper [friend] were here today, welcoming us home. Mum had blown up sixty balloons. Katrina had printed 'Welcome Home Sophie' signs. Jenny and Margaret [Barter] were nurses today and they fitted into the family well. It is just so lovely to relax in the lounge.

Carolyn's journal, Day 187, Tuesday 22 June 2004
A great day at home. Sophie slept till 11 am, so we completed her dressing change at 1 pm – we did not do two today as a result of that. It was busy, with Nadia and a nurse then a changeover nurse. Louise came and entertained Sophie, who was fairly demanding and wanted to sit on my knee a lot.

Sophie struggled with her splints, so woke every hour till midnight. I removed the auxiliary splint and she slept well, waking but being settled by the night nurse, so I got seven hours, which was wonderful. Sophie has handled all the people coming and going well. I still find it difficult thinking what can be done about dinner preparation and baths and getting Mitchell to bed. I'll arrange things better in time, delegate more tasks and encourage Soph to spend more time away from me. It will be good for her and for me too.

Carolyn's journal, Day 188, Wednesday 23 June 2004

We left home at 9 am to go to hospital and got back home at 3.15 pm. It was a full day and that was really pushing it, just to get the bath done and plasters on. I think Sophie was a bit worried we were going to stay at the hospital and was quite relieved when we headed home.

We ran out of time to meet the team at Arranounbai School, so we will do that tomorrow. Carrie from Clubbe Ward called me into her office to say how good it was working with us in 'shared care' and how the nurses will all miss us a lot. She wants to arrange an official going-away party and have Peter Hayward attend.

Sophie is still waking a lot at night and she says things like 'I want to hurt you, Mummy – don't don't don't!' when she is having a bad dream. We are making headway with routines: it would be much better if we had unpacked more fully but we need to clean out before we can put away. Ron is getting impatient about bears being everywhere. It is truly wonderful to have Sophie home.

Carolyn's journal, Day 189, Thursday 24 June 2004

I had a meeting in the morning, so thank goodness Catherine came over to entertain Sophie with the nurse. She did painting and puzzles until it was dressing-change time and sorbolene time. Then lunch and we headed to Arranounbai School, where we spent the afternoon.

Mitchell headed off to rugby with Grandma. Sophie was overtired and temperamental at the school but the set-up is great. She can attend a kindy class and have physio, OT and nursing care on site. The nurse there, Maxine, worked at Westmead for five years and was on the Burns ward, so she can do a dressing change for Sophie, as well as assisting with her range of physio movements while at play – she has twenty exercises to get through each day. We will still have a physio come to the house.

Soph got to ride on a motorised bike and it was wonderful. She cheered right up because she could be independent and go anywhere she liked in the playground. I feel really good about Sophie being there.

Carolyn's journal, Day 190, Friday 25 June 2004
Aiming to leave at 9.30 am for the hospital saw us in the car at 9.50 and without petrol, so a stop at the garage meant we were ten minutes late. Lyn arrived and the nurse helped out at the bath, which meant we went straight up to physio and had time to spare to chase up a number of matters at a much more unhurried pace. I left Lyn and Alison the nurse with physio and had some time for coffee; back home by 3.15 pm.

We had some playtime till nurse Sue arrived. She made Sophie necklaces and bracelets and entertained her till bedtime. Sophie had an unsettled time till midnight and woke on about three occasions with a vomit in the early hours. She was up early at 7.30 am and happily played with [nurse] Jenny in the lounge until her feed lines were twisted.

Carolyn's journal, Day 191, Saturday 26 June 2004
Ron off to golf. Jenny spent time with both Mitchell and Sophie, which allowed me to put a few more things away. Ron bears my grumbling about all the bags in bags still around. Grandma, Margaret [Henry] and Jenny took Sophie off for a walk so Mitchell and I could spend an hour together. It was lovely; we had a pirate picnic in his room.

When Sophie came back, we unpacked some of her clothes. We did a head-dressing change and Jenny [Berry] came to do physio – she used a whoopee cushion and the Peking duck [a soft toy] to do exercises. Next week, I'll really concentrate on Sophie's physio regime. All AINs [Assistants in Nursing] should have read the exercise regime and should be able to help me. I'm not feeling as overwhelmed as I was but still cry and want more than anything for Sophie to be happy.

Carolyn's journal, Day 192, Sunday 27 June 2004
Still getting up in the night – been five nights out of seven.

Ron yells at me where is the plaster/mobile/whatever?

Ron hasn't done any of Sophie's care since we were home. I asked him to get up on Friday night and said, 'Your turn.'

I took off one hour early to drop into Beth's before picking Bec up at the airport. First time I had timeout. Felt complete lack of joy and guilt at being out. Ron says, 'I'm off to the club and to golf.'

[Later.] Sophie went for a walk today with Sharon, which gave me a break to unpack a little. Grandma Joy, Linda and Lillie came over, and Ray and Anita [neighbours from Baranbali Avenue]. I left early to drop into Beth's before picking up Bec at the airport. Ron was not impressed about me leaving without a dressing change being done. We'll have to talk about shared workloads on the weekend, particularly if he golfs on a Saturday. It was great to see Bec. I told Mitchell I was going to the airport to pick up Bec and he said, 'Go now! Go now!'

He had a lovely time at a pirate party at Shelley Beach. We were interviewed by the *Sydney Morning Herald* about Sophie being a miracle, our belief in God and Mary MacKillop. Sophie is demanding and frustrated but she plays well at times with the nurses, particularly if I am out of the room. Overall, she appears happy to be home. Mitchell is really happy we are all together, though he says it is tough watching her frustration.

Carolyn's journal, Day 193, Monday 28 June 2004

Hospital visits scheduled; I aimed to leave at 9 am but we were away at 9.25. It takes that length of time to get Sophie into the car. We have a suitcase on wheels that is always full for our trips to and from the hospital. We were back at 3.30 pm. That was wasting no time at the hospital, though we did have about an hour for lunch to encourage Sophie to eat more food orally. Lyn was great – we got through pain-management meetings, physio, bath, pharmacy and a visit to the volunteers in that time.

Carolyn's journal, Day 194, Tuesday 29 June 2004

We went to Bear Cottage at 11 am, after I had dropped Mitchell off at kindy. I dropped another box of Sophie's clothes off [with friends]; her whole wardrobe is inappropriate for her now. I haven't been able to give away all her shoes, though. Bear Cottage are happy to have a bear museum. I will approach Stella Maris [College] for their input. Louise [Palmer] has been very involved as well.

We arrived back in time for Janet [Pickering] to do physio, then we had Carolyn and Charlotte visit. Mary called in also, so plenty of faces floating through the house and encouraging Mitchell to draw and read and do puzzles. Bec is wonderful with him – she is so confident with young kids and will make a great mum one day. She has taken over where Mum left off, organising Mitchell's breakfast, clothes, baths; it is a huge help.

We continue to have new home nurses who need to be trained; it is getting tiring, so I hope we are getting to the end of it.

Carolyn's journal, Day 195, Wednesday 30 June 2004
A full-on day at hospital again. Anticipated leaving at 9.30 am but actually got away at 9.40 – getting more organised. After the bath and plastering, we had lunch and meetings with OT, PR, volunteers and X-ray, leaving hospital at 3 pm. Knees look okay.

We were late getting back and Katy asked to come over with Olivia and Melissa and Ben. Ben and Mitchell played rugby outside and then Jenny arrived for physio. Sophie did well, with a team of people coaxing her on. Beth arrived, then Lee and Mark and Craig Riddington and, a bit later, Rebecca – we had a wonderful roast cooked, which was fantastic. It's just amazing having our friends' support – it helps ease the burden. By X-ray time, I had had enough of my daughter crying and being distressed, so it helped to cheer me up.

Carolyn's journal, Day 196, Thursday 1 July 2004
I left Sophie with her carer Jenny today. Michelle the physio was with her and also Maxine, the nurse at Arranounbai. Michelle did really well and had her rolling on a large red ball – tummy time. I went to gym with Becs and Michelle, then came home and drove to hospital for dressing change. Meeting with Peter Hayward and then a party, which the hospital put on to acknowledge the fund-raising we had done. Peter indicated that, from now on, we will call the shots with Sophie's health care and healing. The next graft is due the first week in August and may well be an overnight or two-day stay in hospital.

The party was lovely, with NETS, PICU, North Shore and Clubbe Ward staff and volunteers. John Harvey and Peter Hayward said some very nice words and we were presented with a certificate and bear for our fund-raising efforts. John Harvey acknowledged Sophie and Molly, the parents and Mitchell and Lilly's effort in getting the girls home. Mitchell puffed out his chest and went and stood next to Lilly, as proud as punch.

Carolyn's journal, Day 197, Friday 2 July 2004
It's tough: four days of dressing changes, seeing your daughter cry; splinting with plaster, seeing your daughter cry; splints at night, seeing your daughter cry. I have been on the verge of tears since Wednesday. Sophie has taken to saying 'go away, Mummy, go away' during the day and I find it hard to think I will need to do Sophie's plasters, which will inflict more pain on my beautiful little girl. She is happy today, which is lovely: I love seeing that sparkle back in her character. But I can't help but wonder about the emotional toll of her care on me.

Carolyn's journal, Day 198, Saturday 3 July 2004
Went to be photographed at Mary MacKillop Chapel for the *Sydney Morning Herald* article. Sister Bridget was there. Mitchell and Sophie were really good, and Sister Bridget spent some time explaining the carvings on the altar. We had to rush back home, as Ron had jobs to do!

Carolyn's journal, Day 199, Sunday 4 July 2004
We headed off to [friend] Smithy's place for a farewell thank

going home

you to the Woods and to all who arranged the golf day at Manly. It was a lovely day and was my second social activity after leaving hospital. My first was the Humpty Dumpty dinner, where I cried on leaving the house, cried on arriving at the venue, cried during the evening but enjoyed myself none the less. It was never going to be easy the first time I left Sophie, wherever it was going to be.

Carolyn's journal, Day 200, Monday 5 July 2004
Left at 9.30 am for hospital, back at 3.30 pm. We had a picnic lunch to encourage Sophie to eat. Met the dietician. If Sophie doesn't increase her weight, we may have to put more calories into her feeds.

Carolyn's journal, Day 201, Tuesday 6 July 2004
A day at home. We had a *Women's Weekly* interview. Louise, Catherine, Beth and Tully came by. Sophie did really good work on the ball in physio with Robyn, whom she had not met before. We then had a photo shoot with the Woods before their departure for the UK. It was a huge day. In between, I manage to do dressings and feed the family.

Carolyn's journal, Day 202, Wednesday 7 July 2004
We have been given a two-night stay at Quay West [hotel, near Sydney's Circular Quay], so today we are heading off to a holiday in the city. First, though, to hospital for a dressing change and bath, then a meeting, which will be held fortnightly from now on. *Women's Weekly* did a photo shoot at physio,

so we did not do any plastering ourselves. Arrived at the hotel at 4.30 pm. It was wonderful. We had Linda, Wayne and Lillie over, so it was a really late night for Mitchell. Wayne and Ron were watching State of Origin. We had pizza for dinner.

Carolyn's journal, Day 203, Thursday 8 July 2004
We had a day at Sydney Aquarium arranged, then off to the Pavilion on the Park [in the Domain] for a meal. They gave us a wonderful basket full of goodies. Charli from Hi-5 came to surprise Sophie and Mitchell. Sophie sat on Charli's knee and sang 'Ready or Not (Hide Your Eyes)', then we walked back to the hotel. Jenny and I did a dressing change. Mitchell, Bec and Ron headed off to the movies, and I tried to get Soph off to bed at 7 pm. She fell asleep at 8 pm, hopefully for a better night after an unsettled one last night.

Carolyn's journal, Friday 30 July 2004
Soph broke her leg in physio on Wednesday. She was in a kneeling frame; there was a snap. The bone had simply broken. [Because of her long confinement to bed, Sophie had developed osteoporosis.] Dr [Helen] Chriss [the Delezio's GP] looked at it yesterday but we agree that it should be checked with an X-ray at the hospital.

I was feeling vulnerable about our return visit next Tuesday and concerned about Soph's leg; the X-ray results showed a fracture that would normally be treated with pins or traction but they can't do that in Sophie's case [due to the osteoporosis and the risk of infection]. She has her leg in a partial plaster splint, when it should have been operated on. I was in tears – thank goodness Lyn and Lisa were there with me.

Ron came over and we decided to take Sophie home. It is our first major setback since we have been home and it hurts – brings back a flood of emotions. Much like going back to hospital is like stepping back into PICU from Clubbe Ward. Ron has been angry and in tears this afternoon, and Mitchell is on a sleepover, not understanding why we had to go back into hospital. It is like being put through the wringer – there is a drained feeling within you.

My seven-day-a-week, twenty-four-hour-a-day job is challenging, exhausting and satisfying all in one. I thank goodness that I had kindergarten teacher training and an interest in special needs. It seems ironic that I always felt that once I retired, I would become a ward granny. Lyn has been a godsend as our ward granny and I will miss her once she is gone in August. The past three weeks have been a continual challenge to fit in Sophie's care regime with our time constraints. The fact is that we need more time in the day, more hours to do all that is ideal, but we push on, trying to be more efficient, for Sophie's sake. We continue to support the media in fund-raising for hospitals and burns units in Australia and New Zealand as our way of paying back and making a difference. The emotional challenges are ever present but we all try to move forward for Sophie's sake. I'm thankful that Mum and Dad are here to help support Mitchell, because he has missed out on so much. He is having behavioural issues, which we are working hard to address.

Carolyn's journal, August 2004 [no exact date]
I lie here listening to my daughter scream in the next room. My son, husband and mother are away on a family holiday in Bali, where we should have all been together – look at my fragmented family. I try to see the positive but freely admit I would love to be there with them. We talked to Mitch about this being

a special holiday for him before he goes to school next year. Mitchell is suffering a bit at the moment, saying, 'I do not feel delightful when no one is with me at bath time,' and, 'When I go on holiday, my heart will still be here.' It's just terribly sad. I've been in to Sophie three times in the last thirty minutes and she is still distressed as I try to get some sleep.

I've been tearful a lot lately as we try to create some normality in our lives. We've dropped a day at hospital, so at last it seems possible to create some much-needed free time, while still incorporating Sophie's physio needs.

In September, Sophie makes a huge step forward in every sense, when she starts wearing her prosthetic legs that have been custom made for her. 'She was almost running before I could slow her down,' says prosthetist David Hughes.

Carolyn's journal, Wednesday 29 September 2004
A huge week in Sophie's life. Last Wednesday, shoe shopping with Linda. On Thursday, swimming hydrotherapy at hospital; it was a joyous moment. She was so happy in the pool with Ron and Jo [Newsome], and it all came back quite naturally to her.

Friday, we went to a much-needed counsellor. It proved too hard to see Sandra; hospital days are so busy. By the time I organise Mitchell and Sophie, it often absorbs my last available time. I said to Sandra that I will keep her updated with our progress with Ann, but we all agreed that we were still just in survival mode. On Friday, Sophie pulled her tube out. We have been fine-tuning medications and how they are administered; it's not easy on a screaming three-year-old. I have reduced midday meds to nil and fine-tuned others to manage in smaller syringes that are easier to get in her clamped mouth.

We had free tickets to the movies on Saturday, which was fun; achieving one activity with all the medical stuff fills the day. There is still no rest time.

Monday – Sophie's appetite improves with no tube, so we agree with dietician to continue and monitor with no tube.

Tuesday – Sophie ate carrot for the first time since December. She also slid on her prone board, propelling herself inside for the first time. Each day, there are firsts; even if they are small, they mean she is achieving. She is bottom-shuffling well and will move between rooms. She is also wheeling between rooms again now that she has her wheelchair back [it was sent away for adjustment].

Because of holidays, Tuesday and Wednesday were two play days in a row, with only daily physio and meds, bath, etc., which was wonderful. Mitchell and I spend time together on Fridays now, because I feel he has missed so much.

I still lack 'joy', the enthusiasm for life. It is too much to keep a daily log/diary. By the evening, I am physically and emotionally drained.

Carolyn's journal, Tuesday 2 November 2004
I look at the last date and feel that Sophie has achieved so much in the last month. Hydro and new legs; three weeks to arrange the rehab plan, today being the last day of putting it all into practice. Sophie is gaining mobility every day, along with confidence and independence. Even with the new legs, it is an ongoing monitoring issue. Today, talking with Dr Jenny Ault, it appears that we may have a lymph-drainage issue, so she is doing a full review.

I went to the Roundhouse today – a sad and lonely drive. Ron was not able to meet me because of the launch of the Day of Difference Foundation, so I met with Sandra Spalding alone. It was outdoor time and the children were having lunch, so I could walk the path along which the car travelled. I don't think I'll ever find out how a car can turn ninety degrees after clipping a lamp post, drive through two windows airborne and land such a distance from its initial impact with the building. I understand from Sandra that a piece of furniture was propping up the car, so it didn't lie completely on Sophie. Dr Peter Maitz [Concord Hospital] said, though, that Sophie's back was damaged from contact burn, not flame – most likely the heated metal of the fuel tank. All I wanted to do was sit down on the spot where Sophie had been sleeping and have a really good cry. I talked with Janet and cried with Liz [Roundhouse staff]. Both Laura and Amanda have now left, unable to cope with the daily reminder of events – both are on stress leave. There was a peaceful calm about the place, as there always was – just a reminder of what could have been.

Today, Soph did her first hydro session at Arranounbai and swam with floaties and a ring. She also had her first shower, sitting in a special shower chair before and after the pool. She loved it. Her legs had to be adjusted due to swelling, additional weight and oedema.

I walked Mitchell to school and picked him up; it's a small amount of time but very precious to have with him.

Carolyn's journal, Thursday 20 January 2005
I feel like it's been an age since I put pen to paper. It's not for not wanting to but often I'm so tired at night and just want to chill out.

Soph went to theatre yesterday for the start of her elective procedures. Both hands were to be grafted and there were tears all round. At breakfast yesterday, Soph took Ron's hand and then mine and just looked each of us in the eye in a very knowing way. Sophie managed surgery well and her recovery was the best. She's been waking only intermittently and settling quickly. She is quite angry at times, saying 'go away' to nurses and me. She enjoyed seeing Lisa, who changes her behaviour immediately, and she wanted to sleep over a second night so she could see Lyn South [her ward granny].

Soph was weaned off morphine by 11 am and is now only on paracetamol with codeine. She has a really high pain threshold as a result of her previous injuries. Peter will take down her dressings for a bath next Tuesday under a general anaesthetic and we will be back again on Thursday.

It takes a step backwards to move forwards. It is a sad, anxious time of reflection but we have absolute faith in Peter Hayward. I still have waves of a heavy, tight heart – Ron has trouble sleeping. Mitchell had a sleepover at Charlotte's, freeing up our time to be with Soph tonight. She just wanted to be on my lap. The holidays are nearly over and I wonder where the time has gone, eaten away somewhat by physio five days per week. People's daily support still lifts me and I pray to God to give me strength and to guide me.

chapter sixteen
lightning strikes twice

On 5 May 2006, two years and five months after the Roundhouse fire, Sophie is on her way home from school. Rebecca [Bec] Myhre, Carolyn's god-daughter, who is staying with the Delezios and helping to look after Sophie before moving to the UK, has picked Sophie up in her stroller. At the pedestrian crossing on Frenchs Forest Road, Bec brings Sophie's companion dog, Tara, to sit beside her as they wait for a break in the busy afternoon traffic. Cars stop to let them cross; Bec steps out, not seeing that a car in the far lane is not going to stop. Sophie's stroller is hit and flung twenty metres across the road.

Sophie is stabilised with some difficulty by paramedics and taken by helicopter to Sydney Children's Hospital at Randwick, in Sydney's inner east. She has nine broken ribs, punctured lungs, a broken jaw, a broken collarbone, brain injuries and spinal fractures.

Once again, Sophie's life hangs in the balance. Once again, the family is thrown into life-and-death conversations, Emergency waiting rooms and the cold sweat of not knowing.

That such a thing could happen to Sophie a second time defies belief. It is one of those events – like Princess Diana's death, like John Lennon's – that people look back on and remember exactly where they were when they heard the news. This is particularly true of those who know Sophie – but, by this time, all of Australia feels that they know Sophie. The community have drawn her to their hearts and she has become 'Australia's angel', a symbol of hope prevailing against circumstance.

For Sophie's family, though, there has been so little reprieve after the first accident that they simply swing into the old rhythms: organising the roster of friends to sit with them; making meals; answering messages; looking after Mitchell; asking the right questions of the doctors; bringing favourite toys and special mementoes to hang by Sophie's bed; issuing a media statement; calling for prayers; taking up the bedside vigil. And waiting.

Neither Ron nor Carolyn keeps a journal until nearing the end of Sophie's stay in Intensive Care. Their record of the days immediately after Sophie's second accident is drawn from Ron's later reflections and the email updates that Carolyn and her brother Greg send to family and friends around the world.

> From: Carolyn Martin
> Date: Friday 5 May 2006, 2.00 am
> We need your prayers now more than ever.
> http://www.smh.com.au/news/national/burns-toddler-sophie-hit-by-car/2006/05/05/1146335916551.html
> While we deeply appreciate everyone's thoughts and prayers, please don't try the phone lines, as we need to leave them open to find out news on what is happening.
> Love to you all,
> The Martin Family

Ron's journal, Friday 5 May 2006

Well, here we are again. We just can't believe it, that such a beautiful little girl has got to go through this all over again. It made me think, what have I done wrong in this life? Is this some sort of punishment that is causing all of this to happen? I just feel so hurt, so sad. I could hardly bear looking at Sophie for the first time after the accident; I just felt that I've let her down, that I haven't been a good-enough parent . . . I'm just so sad for Sophie. She's my beautiful baby and now she's hurt again.

It was around 4.10 pm and I got a call from Rebecca, Carolyn's god-daughter, who was taking care of Sophie. She was on her way back from the shops to our home, crossing the pedestrian crossing, and she told us that Sophie had been hit by a car. She was in hysterics; I had to talk to someone else at the time, but I was so angry – all I knew then was that a helicopter from Careflight had been called to Sophie's accident and taken her over to Sydney Children's Hospital at Randwick. We were at an architects' meeting at the time, working out the best design for our new home [that we had decided to build] to meet Sophie's needs for the rest of her life, so getting that phone call just numbed us.

All the way in the car to the hospital, we were both in tears. We arrived at the hospital and we were still in tears. I remember Carolyn being in front of me going around to Emergency and there were all these journos and photographers and television cameras focused on us, and Carolyn yelled out, 'Please pray for our little girl.'

We had to wait a little while before we could go in and see Sophie. That is just such an agonising wait: there's nothing to look forward to here. Again, she was put into an induced coma. She didn't look too bad. She had her head bandaged up and a smaller team of medical staff around her compared with the first time: then it was around twenty people; this time it was eight or so. The main problems with Sophie were all internal, so she had to go through an MRI to see what damage had been done.

We met up with Jonny Taitz, who is head of Paediatrics at Sydney Children's and whom we knew quite well. The doctors came back after the MRI, saying that she had nine broken ribs, a suspected couple of broken vertebrae, a suspected broken jaw (which was confirmed later), a broken collarbone and a lot of internal bleeding through the broken ribs – three of which had actually punctured her lungs. At this stage, they were not too sure if there was any brain injury. So she was in a bad way.

It wasn't too long before the police department contacted us to tell us what had gone on. That was a real turnaround from the first accident, when we virtually heard nothing from the police department the whole of the six months we were in hospital. With this accident, I think they must have had a different team involved, or they realised where they went wrong the first time, but they were right onto it, explaining what had happened, telling us what they were doing.

It wasn't so much an accident; it was an incident – someone did go through a pedestrian crossing without stopping. So it's not an accident any more; this is something where someone's done the wrong thing, compared with the first accident, where the chap had a seizure. I've always thought that if someone has a seizure or a heart attack or whatever and they pass out, then they're not to blame, that it could happen to me, it could happen to anyone. How did this make me feel? Probably for a short time there was a bit of anger involved, but I had to get on with taking care of our daughter again. [The driver, John Sharman, who was eighty-years-old, was placed on an eighteen-month good-behaviour bond and disqualified from driving for twelve months.]

Ron's journal, Saturday 6 May 2006
Because of Sophie's head injury, they are treating her as a spinal patient. She was put into the bed in a fixed position and no

one is allowed to move her. Needless to say, Sophie's on full ventilation – she's in an induced coma until they find out what's wrong with her. I just counted up all the drugs going into Sophie at the moment. Medazolan, morphine – there are ten different drugs being pumped into Sophie to keep her alive.

Sophie's CT brain scan showed bleeding on the brain but at this stage no abnormalities or need for surgery, which is good.

Ann-Louise, Carolyn's sister, who lives in France, flew to Australia on the day of the accident. What a shock she's had: to get into a cab from the airport and listen to the news saying that her niece has been involved in another accident. Just bizarre that something would happen on the very day that she arrives.

Ron's journal, Monday 8 May 2006
We were told that there was going to be a press conference and they asked whether I would mind attending. I remember someone asked the head of Intensive Care whether Sophie was getting the best treatment. I quickly intervened, saying that Sophie's getting the best care possible, which is no different from any other child in that Intensive Care department. And I believe that to be the case: that there's no reason why Sophie should be treated any better or any worse than anyone else. I'm a hundred per cent sure that they do their hundred per cent utmost to save these kids' lives. I'd hate to see that the journo was trying to point towards Sophie being given preferential treatment over other kids. It's not the case at all.

Ron's journal, Tuesday 9 May 2006
Feeling really alone again and a little bit 'woe is me', I suppose. Just went for a walk around the hospital; I went near the front

lightning strikes twice

253

door and saw all this press waiting out the front, and we saw a number of candles being lit at the front of the hospital; they were making a shrine for Sophie and I just broke into tears. The love and the care that people are showing for Sophie, it is just absolutely incredible.

We're having a few problems at the parents' hostel. One particular family go out to the pub, by the sounds of it, and come back late, pretty drunk – and they've got their child in Intensive Care. It's something I've never seen before. That people would go out and party like that while their child is in Intensive Care; you're only in Intensive Care if the child's life is at risk. How can you just go out and get drunk and come back and make a disturbance so no one can sleep? I had to call on the hospital staff to quieten them down because it's just not fair. There are a number of other families in the hostel – we need as much sleep as we can get; we need to be as aware and refreshed as we can be to cope with what's going on. I just can't understand some people.

Ron's journal, Wednesday 10 May 2006
Today, we kept on talking to Sophie as though she was still awake, not giving in to the fact that she was in a coma. She opened her eyes every now and then and responded to me, squeezing my hand and nodding – it was just incredible. [It is unusual but not unknown for patients in a medically induced coma to open their eyes and respond to familiar voices.]

I was just about to get in a lift to go to another floor when we heard all this bashing going on inside one of the lifts. The parents who were making all that noise in the hostel were in there, just bashing on the inside of the lift. My God, these lifts are used by parents, by medical staff to move kids up and down floors. They didn't give a damn about what happens, what the results were, what needs to be fixed afterwards. I can't believe there are people around like this.

> From: Greg Martin
> Date: Wednesday 10 May 2006, 5.54 pm
> Dear family and friends,
> Sorry for the lack of update. Things have been a wee bit hectic, to say the least.
> From the start of the week, to be in such a dark, depressing place as a children's Intensive Care Unit, we've come so far. Sophie is a little fighter; she just amazes us all.
> Your emails, calls and thoughts have been amazing and uplifting to us all; they are simply overwhelming. I'm sorry if I can't get back to you all one by one, but, rest assured, all your thoughts and messages get passed along.
> Sophie has kept battling and every day gets a little stronger. She just needs to fight off the infections and she should be okay. She's opened her eyes twice; she even managed to squeeze her dad's hand today. As she improves, so do Caro and Ron and their spirits, which lifts everybody else up. If they can keep going, the rest of us surely should be able to.
> Sophie has been looking better every day as well. Still a little touch and go, but certainly the news gets better every day, rather than worse.
> Please keep the prayers and support coming; they are needed.
> Love to you all,
> The Martin Family

Ron's journal, Saturday 13 May 2006
What an absolutely magical day. Today, we had Danny Green come in, the world-championship boxer. He's been a mate for a little while, since the first accident. I said to Danny, 'Go over the other side of Sophie and I'll take a photo of you.' Danny got

behind the bed and I said, 'C'mon, Soph, smile for Daddy so you can have a photograph with Danny Green.' And we saw a smile on Sophie's face, and she reached back to hold Danny's hand. She's still in an induced coma, but she knows enough about what we're talking about and reaches back with a beautiful smile on her face. I took some photographs, and Danny and I absolutely bawled after that. We thought, man, this is a magical moment; we could not believe what had happened.

From: Carolyn Martin
Date: Sunday 14 May 2006, 12.06 am
Dear friends and family,
Keep the prayers, thoughts and messages coming: they are working. Good news from Sophie's doctors, who say that her injuries are now not life-threatening. The risk of infection is now her only life-threatening concern.
They are going to keep her sedated but have begun reducing the amount of the medicines that are keeping her under, and she is responding to questions by nodding her head and moving her arms. They will keep her under for at least the next two weeks, to allow the broken bones to heal.
She seems a little more comfortable now, as the breathing tube was removed from her mouth (which she always hated) and is now up her nose.
Last night, she even poked out her tongue at Ron when he was tickling her.
Love to you all,
The Martin Family

Ron's journal, Sunday 14 May 2006
They're continuing to wean Sophie off morphine and Medazolan and all those other drugs, so she's slowly starting to come

around a bit more. What we don't really know still is how much damage has been done to her brain. We're still monitoring her movements and continually asking questions as she slowly comes out of her induced coma, making sure she's answering the right way.

Around two o'clock in the morning, I decided to go outside for a bit of a wander around, to stretch my legs and clear my head. I walked around to the front of the building and again noticed that there are candles everywhere, signs and cards saying 'We love you, Sophie' and 'God bless you, Sophie' and 'God will take care of you'. It's hard to believe that so many people care for and love Sophie and are feeling some of the pain that she's going through. But as I walked out the door, I noticed a journalist jump out of his car with his camera in hand and run towards me. I said to him, 'Listen, pal, not now.' And he just turned to me, nodded his head and said, 'No worries, Ron.' Then he went back to his car and drove off. We're getting quite a relationship with the journalists, the newspapers and the media, and quite a respect. They have got a job to do, and if they don't do their job, they haven't got a job to go back to. So I've got to respect that.

On 17 May, Carolyn takes up her journal once more to trace their steps through this new crisis in their lives.

Carolyn's journal, Wednesday 17 May 2006
It's now twelve days after the accident. Two days since I stepped out of the hospital for the first time, only to receive a call from the registrar at ICU, which sent my blood draining and adrenalin rushing.

I reminisce as we walk through these doors and wards again; once again, we are greeted by another family's loss, following an accident the previous afternoon. The emotions weigh heavily and as Sophie loses her sedation the real work for me begins: showing loving support, care and understanding as she is weaned off her drugs and talking through medical matters to ease her pain and anguish in readiness for her rehab to begin.

We have managed these last days relying on our usual back-up team, who have stepped right back into the routine created last time. There has been absolute support from my family: Ann-Louise (France) and Gregory (US), Ma and Pa (New Zealand); unbelievable support from the community, for which we say a huge thank you; and somewhat mixed media messages.

Today, there was a press conference saying that Sophie is smiling at Mum, yet all I recall are the tears and confusion and pain and suffering my child endured today. Actually, I do remember the smile, for it was a precious moment. It was made even more special as Mitchell was holding her hand. I have read hundreds of messages today and am humbled by the love and support our family has, and I take a very serious view of sharing that as best I can.

Carolyn's journal, Saturday 20 May 2006
Out of ICU yesterday – what a day! Dressings and bath and pack up room, then by twelve noon we were on the move. We settled in, along with four boxes of mail; the room was overflowing with people and things.

Back in a ward and adjusting to the different nursing regime. On the one hand, I wish I was back at Westmead, with all the familiarity of the nursing care and the environment; on the other, I'm glad we haven't moved Sophie. I'm calling her home nurses back in on a more full-time basis to help me lift, toilet, wash and dress her. The ward nurses have other care duties and sometimes it's hard just to get a pan! I have to remember to drive what Sophie's needs are and re-establish a routine for Soph, including daytime rest from 12 to 1.30 pm.

We have had a day full of visitors today and I was not able to utilise their talents fully because the room was not organised enough, but they were a good distraction for Soph and helped her pass the day without too much hassle. We started everything late because I couldn't have a shower or go to the toilet till 10 am – there is only one bathroom for parents. And after that everyone arrived: Louise and cousin, Lee, John and Katrina, the police, Mandy and Margaret [Henry], the health minister and entourage, Mum and Dad, Mitchell, Linda, Wayne, Lillie, Pat, Ron, Mary, Frank, Manuel and Carmen Delezio.

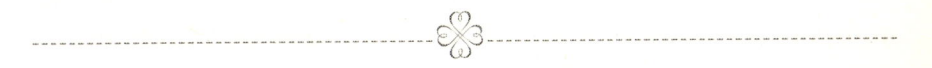

Carolyn's journal, Sunday 21 May 2006
What a night and day – juggling meds, vomits, temper tantrums, X-rays, medical teams. There are such huge expectations on a little girl. X-ray confirmed NG tubes in right place, so drugs could recommence. X-ray showed lung was not getting worse. When Sophie says she can't breathe, we think it's because she is in pain and not taking deep breaths. She is so tired. She woke five times last night: once after monitor beeped, then it was poos and wee, vomit, change sheets, pain. NGs out, retape as best we can, all because a feed bag ran dry – it's at those times that can be avoided that you get really cross.

Slowly making headway with the room: only three bags left to sort out. The mail and gifts have been extraordinary. Visitors today: Dave and Tegan [Palmer], John Mangos [from *Sky News*], Scott, Caroline, Lilly, Molly, Mrs Murray and Mrs Duffy [teachers from Sophie's school], Sensei [Sophie's Japanese teacher], Mitch and Jenny [Berry], Danny, Katy, Melissa and Olivia [Gompes].

Sophie went for her first walk in the hall with Olivia, Katy, Danny and Melissa, then she ate a little with Olivia. Yesterday,

Mitch ran onto the field with the Swans – Soph watched on TV and kept saying she saw Mitchell playing. Mitch went to the rugby league today and met the players with Luke Ricketson. He is, however, really sad to have to leave and wants to do a sleepover at hospital. It would be really good, too, as we have two sofa chairs in our room. Hmmmm – the powers that be! I feel so much better when Soph is resting and calm. Dr Peter arrived and we won't plate her skull – just graft her head.

> From: Greg Martin
> Date: Sunday 21 May 2006, 1.18 pm
> Dear friends and family,
> On Saturday, I called Caro at the hospital and she sounded stressed. Not unusual given the circumstances, I thought. Sophie's feeding tube had come out after a restless night's sleep and she was trying to talk Sophie into letting the doctors put it back in. So she decided to let me try:
> 'Sophie, is that you?'
> 'Yep!'
> 'Are you going to let the doctors put the feeding tube back in?'
> 'Nope!' and she giggles.
> I didn't know whether to laugh or cry. Sophie was back!
> While the same fighting spirit that has kept this little angel going was causing Caro a few short-term headaches, what a great problem to have.
> She continues to amaze us all at the speed she is recovering, but maybe we shouldn't be given her nature and the amount of love, support and prayers she has received from around the world.
> She still has another two to three weeks in hospital to let her bones heal, but if you left it up to Sophie she'd be at home right now. As she said, 'I'm sick of the hospital and want to go home.'
> Love to you all,
> The Martin Family

Carolyn's journal, Wednesday 24 May 2006

Last night, I sat with Katrina, clearing the mail. We are up to date for another day – what a relief. Sophie stood on her prosthetic legs for the first time and took four steps. She rode in her wheelchair but later in the afternoon she had a sore back and neck. She had a really unsettled night and a mixed day in terms of energy. We went for two walks but she did not want her legs on.

It looks like the graft is set for Friday and we wait to hear what the plan is after that. It looks like weeks before we are home, as opposed to months; we need to put the rehab team in place to allow us the flexibility at home. The PAU [Physical Ability Unit] from Arranounbai visited today, as did Jenny B and Dr Epps. David Hughes checked Sophie's legs yesterday. Sandra continues to work with Mitchell and Sophie, coming each Wednesday. Ma brings Mitch over, then he goes back to school at lunchtime. His behaviour at hospital at those times tests me and I find myself getting short with him. The focus of the day rests very heavily on Sophie and her needs, and I find it difficult to cope with both. However, he always gets a treat when he comes to hospital. Ron is spending nights with him, which I hope helps.

Carolyn's journal, Thursday 25 May 2006

As I sit at home tonight and ponder my daughter's operation tomorrow, I reflect on what a committed group are doing at the Day of Difference Manly golf day and dinner tonight.

Sophie had a great morning but not such a good afternoon; our timetable hasn't really been established yet. The best we could do was stretches and physio. The most exciting event: two walks down each end of the hall, one to sing songs and the other to buy something from a vending machine.

Sister Bridget rang, and Nanu, Nana and Adam [Ron's nephew] visited. Firefighter Wade Laverick came by, as did students from the Japanese school with a thousand paper cranes. [An ancient Japanese legend says that anyone who folds a thousand origami cranes will be granted a wish, such as long life or recovery from illness or injury.] Lee arrives with a meal and the secretarial-school volunteers to do all the mail. I've just found out that Sophie hasn't had any meals (or paracetamol) since 11 am; her line was off from 12 until 2 pm, so she had no morphine for two hours. No wonder she didn't want to do physio – although she very rarely complains of pain. Soph is vomiting a lot, so we are having periodic rests from feeds, particularly before meds. Working with new nursing staff is a challenge and I often think it would be easier to be at Clubbe Ward, although our rehab and orthopaedic teams are good here.

I found it difficult to cope with Mitchell yesterday; there are behavioural issues that need to be addressed. Katrina helped me with more paperwork tonight and brought chocolate cake!

Carolyn's journal, Sunday 28 May 2006
I feel a lot calmer and mildly euphoric. Our stay is coming to an end and it's now just the logistics of a home-based care plan. I'm also scared. I went home last night for Mum's birthday, picked up pizza and during the wait felt that familiar feeling of the moment being surreal and lacking in any real meaning. I had the awful realisation that I have to drive over that pedestrian crossing daily, and the sensation of wondering when the joy will come back into our lives. I was the scared, lonely parent of a child having an operation on Friday, hoping that all would go well. Laying trust in the hands of the surgeons and anaesthetic staff and feeling that I wanted to take all of the fear and pain away from my little girl as she waited to go into theatre. I held her in my arms and lay next to her during her anaesthetic. Peter was happy and Sophie made a great recovery. Yesterday,

she was a little teary and didn't want me to leave. Today, she surprised us all by moving herself up the bed and eating two cups of chicken-noodle soup – broth only, but it's a start. She is being weaned off the morphine, and larger pockets of our precious little girl are visible.

Carolyn's journal, Tuesday 30 May 2006
Today Tonight aired last night and was well received, by all accounts. The days are so busy, they just fly by. We are now in the rehab-planning phase, looking at the possibility of being home within the week. OT have done an equipment review; the school is looking at timetables. Our home-based physios came in to do a review with Margaret from physio. Dr Epps checked Soph and met with Toni Blanch [Sophie's case manager]. Brett Kirk from Sydney Swans visited again; he has been in each week. Soph put her legs on and kicked a whoopee cushion to him and reached really high with a stretch like the players. This afternoon with Jen [Jenny Berry] and Robyn and Margaret, she played the guitar with [music therapist] Fiona – Mitch on drums. Soph in legs with headphones and a *Bananas in Pyjamas* crown that Mitch made – quite a sight!

Soph is off the morphine and is trying small amounts of a variety of foods on offer. She had the most delightful time opening all the gifts she has been sent. We will find a good home for them all. Each gift offers a small distraction to a little girl who is only allowed to venture to the vending machine or the covered walkway on level three as an escape from her room. Tomorrow, ABC Kids/*Playschool* will be in to do a concert, and she's really looking forward to it. She keeps asking when the Wiggles will be coming in!

Carolyn's journal, Thursday 1 June 2006
Sophie loved the *Playschool* concert and was allowed for the first time to venture to level nought [of the hospital]. She woke asking when it would be on – she really wanted to hurry the morning along.

Fiona (music therapist) has been fantastic. Schoolwork is not a huge focus yet. Today, Soph had a fantastic session with sound waves, physios, OT and Fiona. She used her legs to make synthesised music, then she had a little concert. After that, she was enthused to put legs on and go to level nought. We walked up to admissions and visited Harold the giraffe. Soph chose a lamington at the cafe but did not eat it – food is still a major issue, as everything does not taste quite right. At least she is willing to try. Dr Epps has suggested a small test to see if that part of the brain has been injured, which is worthwhile.

I am feeling the effects of continuous broken sleep. Not as sharp with things – forgetful. Fortunately, Katrina was in today to help finish off the mail, get me dinner, etc. Sophie wanted to sit in the wheelchair and feed herself soup as Katrina and I had dinner; it was a dinner party and Sophie managed well until her elbow and nose started to hurt. We are hoping to get a good block of at least three hours' sleep tonight. It will make all the difference. Sophie has agreed I can sleep over with Mitch on Monday night.

Ron's journal, Thursday 1 June 2006
We've been talking more to Dr Epps and the rehab team regarding discharge and where we see Sophie's brain injury leading. At this stage, it does seem as though there could be some damage to her brain; we're not sure exactly what – we've got to do some more assessment on that. But another worry that has sprung up is that children with this sort of injury are more likely to have seizures or fits in the future. We can only pray that Sophie doesn't have to suffer any more than she already has. It would be absolutely awful after everything that Sophie has been through in her life

to see her having a fit. I'm not sure how I could handle that, let alone how she could handle it, the poor darling.

Carolyn's journal, Saturday 3 June 2006
Sophie had her lines out today and screamed with fear when she saw the blade to be used to remove the stitches. She was okay once it was done and didn't want to talk about what made her scared during the procedure. My poor, beautiful little girl. I tried to shield her eyes but it would have been better had she been in my arms to start with, as we had to stop while I climbed into bed to hold her. She bounced back really well and was very clearly happy that the lines were out.

Today was a happy day, with Magic Maree and Linda visiting. Mitchell and Sophie sat and played in her bed while Ron and Grandma relaxed in chairs. I took a half-hour walk to Randwick shops, looking for Ron's birthday present. This was the first time I had explored outside the hospital in a month. We had gone to dinner with Lee and Mark while Soph was in ICU, which was disastrous. We were only out for an hour. As my main course was placed in front of me, the doctor from ICU rang and my blood rushed from me or adrenalin pumped into me – one or the other. It was a routine call but I immediately panicked and lost my appetite.

It's 9 pm now and our bedtime. My feet hurt and I'm really tired but excited to be going home soon.

Carolyn's journal, Monday 5 June 2006
We had a great discharge-planning meeting today, with all teams present: OT, physio, plastics, dietician, paeds, Toni, the Noakes [agency] home nurses, rehab. Orthopaedics want X-ray, smell

lightning strikes twice

265

and taste tested. Neuropsych being tested in August. At the end of the meeting, as I caught up with Toni, we saw Sophie eating pizza, which she had made with the play therapists.

After a quick catch-up with Sophie, we did the dressing change in the ward and checked her donor site, which looked good. It was interesting watching the vac dressing system being applied [the dressing has a line on it attached to a vacuum; it speeds up the skin's healing process]. Very fortunately, we had Michelle (play therapist) in to distract Sophie. Then we had lots of distractions with presents. Lisa (play therapist from Westmead) came over, and we had an impromptu party for Dad with Captain Starlight and Anita (physio). Then Lee and Susan Wood [friend from New Zealand] did the mail, for which I'll be forever grateful. We have caught up enough so that we can sort and categorise and box to take home. We were very late getting to bed tonight as we had a late bowl of soup prepared by Lee, which Soph loved. We need to track her input but today is a better day for food – the best day yet. We have been given Thursday as a discharge date, which is fantastic. When I told Mitchell, he wanted to make quite sure that it was a firm date. Slept over last night with him, which was lovely.

Carolyn's journal, Wednesday 7 June 2006

'Don't wait for a light to appear at the end of the tunnel. Stride down there and light the bloody thing yourself!'
Sara Henderson (written on a pillow in the hospital)

It's our last night of what has been a long journey – five weeks at Randwick hospital. With a rehab plan in place, we go home to commence a schedule/routine as busy as the last one was when we arrived home from Westmead. I'm looking forward to it, although I also find it quite disorientating being at home again, even more so assimilating into the community. It's like you are an oddity, with people not knowing what to say or do in front of you.

It's the start of Gold Week for the hospital, so an outside broadcast will occur at the same time as 'Sophie and family' leave the hospital. Lots of media expected. Brett Kirk called in again. We met people from Holden who have done a fund-raiser, and Fairy Sparkle [a special hospital visitor] came; we left some fairies in the garden and we will leave fairies in the treatment room too.

Once again, it will be hard to juggle Sophie's care with an intense little boy who is boisterous and bold and jealous of my time with Sophie, all in one package. I struggle with it from time to time and he gets the short straw.

Ron's journal, Thursday 8 June 2006
Had a good session with Dr Taitz and we're out of the place! So we said our thank yous around the wards and Intensive Care. Much as they did a fantastic job with Sophie, we need to be home; Mitchell needs us to be home; Sophie needs to be home as well – we all need to be home as a family. We were going to wheel Sophie out in a wheelchair but there was absolutely no way. She was going to walk out of that hospital and she told us, 'I want to walk, Dad. I want to walk, Mummy.' We were a bit cautious about it because we knew there was a big media frenzy outside the front doors. There was everyone there from all the radio stations, television stations, newspapers. The CEO of the hospital walked out with us and said how proud he was that Sophie had recovered well and was going home. Then I said a few words. Then they made a walkway in between all the media. We walked through, got in the car and went home, with Scott driving us again. Hallelujah.

In mid-June 2006, Sophie goes back to the Children's Hospital at Randwick for a graft on the back of her head. After her operation, she is moved to a general ward. It's the first time the family have had to contend with the noise and lack of privacy; it is not easy to manage Sophie's post-operative needs in that situation.

Carolyn's journal, June 2006 [no exact date]
I know Mary MacKillop is holding Sophie's hand. Another day in hospital and I realise how important it is to have our own room for private, quiet time when Soph is unhappy after surgery. To be in a crowded six-room ward does nothing for my psyche, either. The regularity of our hospital visits requires a routine that I work hard at maintaining. Not easy in a new hospital and changing wards each time we come out of surgery. We have been put in the day-stay ward of the surgical/heart C2 south; a noisy eleven-year-old keeps mentioning Sophie's second accident, the details of which she is not aware of at this stage. [Ron and Carolyn told Sophie only the most basic facts about her accident after a couple of weeks – she gradually learnt more over the course of her recovery.] The parents/accommodation lounge is filled with sleep-out beds, chairs and cots and has no appeal whatsoever. No one knows when the clown doctors will be in when I ask and all I want is the familiarity and routine of Westmead. It spurs me on to have her weaned off her meds so we can go home tomorrow if possible. I'm not sure where we will be moved to if we have to vacate the bed because of day-stay requirements. The staff seem really friendly and attentive; it seems a happy ward. Dr Catherine [Boorer, plastic surgeon] is happy with the graft, which has a vac pump attached. The dressing will come down again in theatre next week (Tuesday) – no more vac!

chapter seventeen
the long haul

With Sophie, it is hard to talk of 'recovery', as she will never be restored to the full health she enjoyed when she was two. Over the next few years, she will have annual neuropsychological testing to check for any ongoing impact on her brain function. But she is now home again after her second accident, settling back into school, family life and the daily rounds of physio and home nursing.

The second accident still bears its marks on the whole family: Mitchell suffers greatly from separation anxiety during this new crisis, becoming agitated when away from his parents. Even Tara, Sophie's companion dog, who was on the crossing with Bec and Sophie when the accident happened, has become flighty around cars. She has to be retrained to become a reliable companion for Sophie again.

From late 2007, Ron and Carolyn make a conscious effort to 'de-medicalise' their lives. As the gaps between hospital visits grow longer, they start to cut back on the amount of home-nursing care they have for Sophie and work hard to find opportunities for her to *do after-school activities such as drama, just like any other girl. In January 2008, though, a post-operative infection brings all of their old fears for Sophie to the surface yet again.*

Plans for their new home progress. After looking at many houses that proved unsuitable for their needs, Ron and Carolyn have found a block of land in Balgowlah Heights that will lend itself to the 'house for Sophie's lifetime' that they dream of building.

Once again, Carolyn's journal becomes a window onto their 'standout days' and moments of reflection on where their lives have led them.

Carolyn's journal, Tuesday 10 October 2006

I cried yesterday as my beautiful girl said to me she didn't want to have an operation. Up until last night, when we lay together in bed and she said this to me, she had been happily telling anyone who would listen that she was going into Westmead for an operation and just what Dr Peter had in mind for her. She had been so openly confident about it all but it struck me that she is still a little girl who gets scared.

The hurt surfaced for me – I would prefer that she wasn't going in for another operation – and I felt deep sorrow that I can't make it better for her. I can just help her to look at the outcome.

It brought up the last accident as well; it has certainly been more front of mind over the last week. As we address Mitchell's issues of separation anxiety with a psychologist at Randwick, walk with and retrain Tara at the crossing with assistance dogs, meet the crew of Careflight who helped care for our little girl and realise how close she came a second time to dying, we thank God for the marvels of medical intervention and the very dedicated teams who are involved in making change happen.

Once again, Sophie has shown me her incredible strength by heading off to hospital and now, post–op, as I write this by torchlight, I watch her beautiful smile despite the multitude of drains, lines and other paraphernalia coming out of her tiny body. She is settled – a good post-op recovery. The familiarity of Westmead is calming. My beautiful, brave, spirited girl sleeps peacefully and I thank God.

Carolyn's journal, Tuesday 28 November 2006
Another operation ahead of schedule due to an infection; not totally unexpected but frustrating and concerning none the less. We expect a positive result from Peter at the end of it. I fear that one day we may have to relive the horror of the early days, when we did not know if Sophie would make it out of theatre or when complications arose. This memory is heightened as I read the transcript of the book *Sophie's Journey* [Sally Collings, 2007], learning more about what happened and the conflict that remains with some people. It brought up a turbulence of emotions for me.

Sophie has rested well post-op and is now eating cheese balls and Pods with Katrina – they are both giggling and playing games. Katrina is my night-time organiser, always arriving with pen, paper and notebooks. Soph has vomited a lot – a combination of post-op anaesthetic and morphine. She is now singing songs with her Dora doll. I've welcomed Katrina's company because, despite the familiarity of the hospital, there is still a sense of isolation and the realisation that you're here because you have a sick child.

We said hello to all our friends today. The familiar faces make it more welcoming; there's Lisa and the volunteers and Prof [Professor Richard Widmer] the dentist, who has the most wonderful manner, and Kate the anaesthetist, who has performed many operations on Soph.

Carolyn's journal, Wednesday 29 November 2006
A better day today but started off sad, with Soph just crying. I couldn't make her feel better. Dr Peter came in and said he too had been feeling sad. Then, after getting Sophie dressed, sitting her in the chair and giving her a head dressing, she was done by 10 am and off morphine, in the wheelchair and ready to go out for the day. Which is exactly what we did.

Mrs Hawkes, Soph's teacher's aide, came to visit and she got the grand tour that had been well planned by Soph during the morning. Soph was so much happier – she had painting and dough and Lisa and Sandra to entertain her. Distraction and Soph go hand in hand at hospital. We saw some more familiar faces and hospital friends, then Ron came for lunch, and Pat and Mitch came for dinner. We visited the Starlight Room before bed. Sophie is much happier off morphine – no more vomiting and less itching. Her head is patchy but she has gained 3–4 cm of hairline. Infection is a problem but all we can do is wait and see what is to be.

I'm much calmer the day after the op – it's countdown to going home. I think each op brings with it memories of so many ops before. But you meet some amazing families and extraordinary children inside these walls. I hope we give them hope and in some small way make a difference to their day.

Carolyn's journal, Friday 1 December 2006
We could have been discharged last night but I wanted three days of IV antibiotics, especially if Soph fights taking her meds. She had a great night's sleep, her appetite has returned and I'm happy with the plan about her head. It is a pretty graphic wound, so we need to keep Webril on when we are out and about to keep the flies off.

It's always a happy time going home, knowing that things have gone well and that we can tick another op off the list. It will give us a good break over Christmas and New Year, which will be wonderful. I'm excited about the future and hope that next year we can have the break that we didn't get this year.

I spent time talking with the mum in the next room; her daughter Chantelle is sad and in pain. Soph visited too and just had a chat; I hope we helped. We talked about Soph's yoga breathing and imagining a safe and happy place to take her away from where she is: immobile in bed. We just approach things in a particular way and fortunately Soph has the personality to run with it. We are very, very lucky.

Carolyn's journal, Wednesday 21 November 2007
There have been many occasions when I have thought to put pen to paper but time seemed to get in the way or perhaps it wasn't the right time. Although there were still plenty of hospital trips, the last six months have given us the biggest gaps from hospital ever (since 15 December 2003).

Sophie walked into theatre today; she climbed onto the bed, put the strawberry mask to her mouth, closed her eyes and went to sleep. The strawberry masks had been donated from Princess Margaret's Children's Hospital in Perth – they worked a treat. It certainly was the best pre-op we've seen and she has had her calmest post-op period ever, even though she is itchy from the residue of tape remaining over her eyes and mouth and from the morphine. Dr Peter is happy, so everyone's happy.

The spaghetti boscaiola from the cafe upstairs is proving to be a winner – five bowls!

Today, Sophie had a graft on her left ear, a contracture release on her neck, two pins into her arm and finger, which is now in plaster, a staple out of her left hip and donor site on tummy. I have decorated her room with the usual posters and prayers; the bag of lucky charms is attached to her bed and has gone with her every time she is in theatre. I hope we are in for a quiet night. I was really nervous for a couple of weeks before the op, wondering how she would go and reliving past experiences, which were not all pleasant. You never want to see your daughter in pain but we approach it on a matter-of-fact basis and although Soph admits to being a bit scared she is amazingly stoic. While in recovery, she complained that her ear was hurting; the nurse asked if on the pain scale it was number one (the lowest) or number ten (the highest). Soph immediately answered 'eleven' and a bolus of morphine was administered. It made us all smile. She will have some more trips to theatre between now and Christmas but Peter says no pins in for Christmas, which is good.

We have been blessed this year with some amazing opportunities: ambassador to the Sydney Swans; *Sophie's Journey* release; a trip to Perth; trips to Dubai and France, where Sophie's favourite thing was the sleepover with her cousins, while Mitchell's was staying in the desert. In Perth, Sophie loved the pool, Mitch loved the Perth Mint and I just loved being there – the opportunity to travel with Soph while she was medically well has been amazing. It's been a long road and, once we are in the new house, I will feel like this chapter has closed and we can move on; by then, it will have been five years.

Carolyn's journal, Thursday 22 November 2007
I remember one of the doctors saying, 'You should never consider hospital a second home,' but it is like one. When you are back in, it's a chance to renew friendships and continue routines, seek out the good food and explore new areas of the hospital. We will be heading home tomorrow. We just couldn't get the pump off in time for release tonight.

Soph had a wonderful day with Magic Maree. [Ward granny] Lyn called in, as did Joyce [a volunteer at Westmead], her nephew Greg, the clown doctors and Katrina, Ron and Mitchell. Soph and Katrina spent a lovely evening doing girlie things. Robyn kindly brought paints from play therapy. The medical teams had only finished the day's plan and review by 11.30 am, so we were late starting on the exit strategy and Soph was in quite a bit of pain over the ear – not the hand, as Dr Peter had anticipated.

I hope Soph will be happy tomorrow so we can get mobile and walk outside the ward. Great to see so many familiar faces in the nursing staff; it makes for much easier care of Sophie.

I left hospital for the first time ever today without Ron or family being around and went to pick up her Pixie Pushchair [stroller for children with special needs]. Magic Maree was keeping her entertained and Soph was doing her bit with magic tricks. Sandra came and spent some time with us as well. Soph always looks forward to that. I'm okay and looking forward to going home.

In January 2008, Sophie starts to have problems with her legs. Some tissue dies. Seeing the flesh turn black, Carolyn and Ron are filled with a dreadful sense of 'here we go again'. There follow five trips to theatre in a month. Sophie is fitted with vac pumps on both legs to speed up the healing and beat the risk of infection. For two months, Sophie is immobile, and for a further four months she cannot use her legs.

Carolyn's journal, Tuesday 4 March 2008
Soph has just had 3 cm off her legs. Dr Peter happy with op. Soph responded well to the new pain-reduction protocol. This op was the result of two harrowing Thursdays in hospital. The first we were here till midnight, following an infection in her right leg. Clindamycin was used instead of IV antibiotics, which was great – otherwise it would have been a five-day stay on

intravenous drugs. Next review was with Peter, who was keen to have us in within a couple of days to manage the legs. He felt the ulceration would take six months to heal, then rehab – it will be eight weeks till she is on her legs again.

It is different seeing Soph with shorter legs. A little less of her tiny body and she is so brave about it. She walked on her knees to theatre – no pre-med – but she got to the door and started crying. You could see the fear in her eyes. It breaks your heart. I cradled her in my arms and (theatre) nurse Ann talked her through going diving under the sea.

No more than twenty minutes' sleep at a time since 10.30 pm – pain not allowing sleep. Soph has her drip in her right arm, so it is difficult to use; she needs feeding and 'all cares' [teeth cleaning, face wash, body wash, etc.]. She can scratch her own nose, though!

Carolyn's journal, Wednesday 5 March 2008
I'm so tired that my back aches and I had to bribe my way out of scratching Soph for hours on end. The morphine controls her pain but makes her irritable, itchy and sick, so we are always trying to find the balance in pain relief. The second half of the day was better than the first. Soph misses Mitchell terribly; she was crying in the middle of the night for him and crying for him today – I rang Pat and asked her to bring him in. Soph was so happy when he arrived – there were big hugs all round. On departure, however, Mitch got all sad and teary, so I walked with him and Ron up to the main entrance, giving lots of cuddles along the way.

Have arranged OT for Thursday and had Cheri and Sandra check in on Soph. The clown doctors provided a huge amount of entertainment, as did Robyn the play therapist. A little laughter goes a long way and Soph's outlook was more positive from that point on.

Carolyn's journal, Tuesday 25 March 2008
It seems like this has been a long haul, with the three weeks preceding the last op and the last three weeks. Troubleshooting Sophie's pain management, wondering how she got an infection in the first place and now wondering how long till her legs heal. During these times, I get scared of the unknown, of what we haven't experienced in terms of her care. It brings back memories of her acute medical stage, when we went through one crisis after another. While the gaps widen, it is still scary and I pray to God to give me strength to give her strength, and for Dr Peter and the nurses, etc. to help her get well.

I'm lying here listening to the familiar pump of the vac dressing, which drowns out the hum of the air bed, which drowns out the beep of the monitor. I feel quite bruised and battered but know that while Dr Peter hasn't seen legs behave like this before, we are in extremely capable hands. Again, I think of our friends and support team, the ones who have stuck with us and the ones who, disappointingly, we have lost along the way. We consider ourselves very lucky to meet wonderful people who inspire, and we try to help others as best we can.

Carolyn's journal, Wednesday 26 March 2008
I felt as though there was a whirlpool of decisions and treatment today: pain medication, which Soph took willingly without a fight; getting a timeframe for being home; antibiotics following a staph infection; how to pre-medicate for a dressing change on Friday; how to mobilise Soph while at home; review with OT on wheelchairs; meeting with hospital school principal [patients who are well enough can attend school at the Children's Hospital at Westmead]; noting our needs and working with Soph's school and class teacher Ann Murray if she comes to hospital for any length of time (the issue is of

her losing ground scholastically and not being able to make up the time); meetings with social workers to discuss Soph's emotional needs and various issues that have come up; meeting with anaesthetist Reg to plan pre-med strategy for dressing change in theatre or Clubbe Ward; purchase of new pillow from volunteers' shop to help support legs.

By mid-morning, I needed a coffee! And to walk in the fresh air and to make numerous calls to rearrange the week at home, Mitchell's extra-curricular activities, things for Beatrice Street [new house], etc. – and life goes on. We've met two teenagers who are depressed – Sophie's teenage years could be interesting.

Carolyn's journal, Thursday 27 March 2008
Dr Peter has his usual wonderful way of putting things in perspective: so as not to get too hung up on infection, we put things in a larger context. A much smoother day, with a plan hatched for surgery. Soph woke in acute pain at 6 am – no night meds were given. Have to get onto the nurses about that. Settled her down again but need to keep up a regular supply of medication to her today. Claire came over, Sophie's gorgeous carer, whom she loves like a big sister. They had a lot of fun, giving me an hour off for coffee and to organise my day and make the calls that needed to be made.

Volunteers were thanked for their support, particularly Joan for new nighties and Joyce, who found me a shirt from her stall because we stayed in longer than I had clothes for. I had asked Pat, her other carer, in because I thought it important for her to see how to manage Soph's mobility. My aim was also to get her home carers to the hospital school so, if they were with her at Westmead in the future, they would know the routine. I want Soph to have the option of doing work there so she doesn't lose ground on her schoolwork.

Had a laugh with Debbie from PR, who said Soph was so consistent:
1) Call for clown doctors.
2) Request chocolate.
3) Feed fish.

Carolyn's journal, Tuesday 1 April 2008
Back in for a 'little bit of work' by Peter and . . . into Sophie's old room. It's where she had her third birthday and where I hope she doesn't have to have her seventh. It really would be good to get her home tomorrow night so she can wake up on her birthday in her own bed!

Soph was in a lot of pain post–op – a graft onto both legs, the donor site being her thigh. Once we had enough morphine on board, she settled, although she hasn't eaten her usual hearty post-op meal. It's 11.30 pm and the air bed has finally arrived; I hope Soph will now settle to sleep. This must be my fifth time of trying to write – itchy ear, toilet stop, pillows for legs and the hum of the air bed drones on in chorus with the chirping of the vac pump. Let's hope we are over the hurdle and on the mend. Monday will be a dressing change and Soph's fourth trip to theatre in two weeks (just under). It has been a long haul and it absolutely breaks your heart when Sophie asks, 'Why do we have to do it again? We only did it last week.' You can see the fear and anxiety in her eyes before the mask. It's 11.40 pm and she says, 'This bed is really comfy – I'm really pleased – it's way more . . .' and drifts off to sleep.

who's who

All medical professionals and patients were at the Children's Hospital at Westmead, unless specified.

NAME	DESCRIPTION
Adrienne Epps, Dr	rehab specialist, Sydney Children's Hospital at Randwick
Allan Martin	Carolyn's father
Amanda Zimmerman	Roundhouse childcare worker
Amish Vora, Dr	registrar
Amy Gaffey	PICU nurse
Andrew/Andy Williams, Dr	doctor
Angela Holden	PICU nurse
Ann-Louise de la Poype	Carolyn's sister
Anne Lamont	volunteer
Antoni Delezio	Ron's grandson; Catherine's son
Beckie Bateman	PICU nurse
Ben Davis	patient; parents Robyn and Brian
Beth Minogue	friend
Bettina Kolker	PICU nurse
Bridget, Sister	Mary MacKillop Chapel, North Sydney
Captain Starlight	entertainer for sick children
Carmen Delezio	Ron's sister
Carol Inkson	friend
Caroline Wood	Molly's mother
Carolyn, James and Charlotte Reid	friends
Carrie Hopwood	nursing-unit manager, Clubbe Ward
Catherine Delezio	Ron's daughter
Cheri Templeton	physiotherapist

Chris Sharma	friend from New Zealand
Christopher Cooke	friend
Cliff Neville	*60 Minutes* producer
Connie Somers	Clubbe Ward nurse
Craig Riddington	friend; former champion Ironman
Damian Marucci, Dr	plastic surgeon
Dave Palmer	friend
David Binks	friend
David Hughes	prosthetist, Sydney Children's Hospital at Randwick
David Murrell, Dr	anaesthetist
Debra Fowler	public-relations officer
Dee and Carol	friends from New Zealand
Dianne Ward	Clubbe Ward nurse
Dorothy (Dot) Napper	volunteer
Felicity Cooper	friend
Fleur Wood	friend
Frank and Mary Delezio (Nanu and Nana)	Ron's father and mother
Geata Jarrett	Roundhouse director
Gemma Lowe	PICU nurse
Georgia Hammit	friend
Gracie Cooper	patient and friend
Greg Martin	Carolyn Martin's brother
Helen Chriss, Dr	the Delezios' GP
Irene Kopp	PICU nurse
Jan Donohoo	hospital chaplain
Janet Binks	friend
Janet Pickering	physiotherapist
Jeff Fatt	purple Wiggle
Jenny Ault, Dr	rehabilitation specialist

Jenny Berry	physiotherapist, Sydney Children's Hospital at Randwick
Jenny Nickolas	home nurse
Jessica Cooke	Roundhouse friend
Jo Hansen	friend
Joan Cottrell	volunteer
Johanna (Jo) Newsome	physiotherapist
John Delezio	Ron Delezio's son
John Harvey	head of burns
John Mangos	television newsman, *Sky News*
John Stewart	friend from Coffs Harbour
Jonathan Gillis	ICU specialist
Jonny Taitz, Dr	head of Paediatrics, Sydney Children's Hospital at Randwick
Joy Martin	Carolyn's mother
Joyce Duncan	volunteer at the Children's Hospital at Westmead
Jude Gilbert	friend from New Zealand
Justin Cooke	friend
Kam Soon Lim	anaesthetist
Kate Delezio	John Delezio's wife; children William and Oliver
Kathryn McNamara	PICU nurse
Katrina Brayshaw	friend
Katy Gompes	Olivia's mother (Roundhouse)
Kerry Griffin	One of the mums first on the scene at the Roundhouse
Laura Hayman	Roundhouse teacher
Lee Tonelli	friend
Lilly Fay	friend
Lilly Wood	Molly's sister
Lincoln Holmes	*60 Minutes* producer

Linda Jones Meader	friend; husband Wayne, daughters Lillie and Elysa
Lisa Carnovale	play therapist
Liz Hayes	*60 Minutes* presenter
Lorraine Wood	friend
Louise Jennings	PICU nurse
Louise Northcott	paediatrician
Louise Palmer	friend
Lucas Wilkes	patient; mother Sue
Lyn South	ward granny
Mandy Henry	friend
Manuel Delezio	Ron's brother
Maree Thomas	friend; Sophie's 'fairy godmother'
Margaret Barter	home nurse
Margaret Henry	friend
Margaret Maroney	Clubbe Ward nurse
Mark Tonelli	friend; former Olympic swimmer
Mary O'Connor	friend; advised Carolyn on business purchase
Matt Tallis	physiotherapist
Max Dodd	friend
Maxine Amies	nurse, Physical Ability Unit, Arranounbai School
Melissa Cooke	friend; helped with fund-raising
Michael Cooke	Mitchell's friend
Michelle Bates	Ron's sister
Michelle Carne	physiotherapist
Mitchell Delezio	Sophie's brother
Molly Wood	another child badly burnt at the Roundhouse; parents Scott and Caroline, sister Lilly
Nadia Vigna	occupational therapist
Nanu and Nana (Frank and Mary Delezio)	Ron's father and mother

Olivia Gompes	another child at the Roundhouse on the day of the accident; mother Katy
Pam Cheung	Clubbe Ward nurse
Pat Barraclough	home carer
Paul Coleman, Father	Mary MacKillop Chapel, North Sydney
Paul Hammett	friend
Peter Hayward, Dr	plastic surgeon
Peter Maitz, Dr	Concord Hospital burns specialist
Peter Overton	*60 Minutes* presenter
Rebecca (Bec) Myhre	Carolyn's god-daughter
Rebecca Riddington	friend; husband Craig
Rod Smith	solicitor; daughter Mikala
Russell Cherry	old friend; son Aaron, wife Janice
Sandra Spalding	hospital social worker
Sarah Clarke	Clubbe Ward nurse
Scott Wood	Molly's father
Sharon White	play therapist
Siobhan Connelly	Burns Unit clinical-nurse consultant
Susan Farugia	nurse
Therese Conolly	harmoniser
Toni Blanch	Sophie's hospital case manager
Tracey Hammett	friend
Tricia Cummins	PICU nurse
Trudy Wise	friend; helped with media and fund-raising; children Zach and Eleanor Rose
Tully Dodd	friend
Vere Sharma	friend
Wayne Meader	friend

medical terms and abbreviations

Albumin – blood-plasma protein

Arterial line – a thin catheter (tube) inserted into an artery (usually in the neck), used to monitor blood pressure and get samples for arterial-blood-gas measurements

Bactigrass – an antiseptic dressing that soothes injuries such as burns and helps reduce infection and inflammation

BMP – Basic Metabolic Panel: a set of tests that measure the status of the kidneys, electrolyte and acid/base balance, blood sugar and calcium levels

Bolus – a single dose of a drug or other medicinal preparation given all at once

Breakthrough morphine – used to treat severe flares of pain that 'break through' usual pain medications

Broviac line – a type of central line, similar to a Hickman line

Central line – a soft plastic tube that is inserted in a vein in the neck, chest or groin (in Sophie's case, the chest was the most common site) to give fluid and drugs or take blood samples

Chloral hydrate – a sedative drug

Chlorvescent – used to treat hypokalaemia, an electrolyte imbalance common in hospitalised patients

Clindamycin – an antibiotic

Clonidine – lowers blood pressure; also used to treat post-op pain and withdrawal symptoms

CT scan – computed tomography: an advanced form of X-ray that creates a three-dimensional image of the inside of the body

Diazepam – a drug that treats anxiety, seizures and insomnia

ECG – electrocardiogram: a test that checks for any abnormalities in the heart by recording electrical activity

Endocrinology – the branch of medicine that deals with hormones, which regulate growth, development and tissue function

Extubate – remove ventilation and other tubes inserted in the body

Exu-Dry jacket – a special burns dressing

Femoral line – a central line inserted into the femoral vein, in the groin

Hickman line – a type of central line

ICU – Intensive Care Unit

Intubate – insert a tube into a body orifice, such as down the windpipe for ventilation

IV – intravenous, as in the supply of liquids directly into a vein, such as by a drip

Jelonet – a soft paraffin dressing

Jobst – a pressure garment that helps to keep skin grafts intact

Ketamine – an anaesthetic drug

Lavage – washing out the lungs for therapeutic or diagnostic purposes

Linogram – a scan of the central line (done by radiography)

Medazolan – a sedative drug (Medaz for short)

MRSA – Methicillin-resistant *Staphylococcus aureus*: a bacterium that causes difficult-to-treat infection (often referred to in the press as a 'superbug')

Nasogastric tube – a soft tube inserted through the nose, down the throat and into the stomach, used to administer feeds and medication

NETS – Newborn and Paediatric Emergency Transport Service

Nitrous oxide – laughing gas

Oedema – the build-up of internal fluid

Oncology – the branch of medicine that studies cancerous tumours

Ondansetron – an anti-nausea drug

Orthotics – the field of the health-care profession that designs devices to correct muscular or skeletal deformities of the body

Osteomyelitis – an infection of the bone

Osteoporosis – a bone disease that results in an increased risk of fracture

OT – occupational therapy

PICU – Paediatric Intensive Care Unit

Prone – lying face down

Pseudomonas – a bacterium that causes infection

Scarlet red – ointment/dressings used to promote healing of wounds

Supine – lying face upwards

Transpyloric line/tube – a feeding tube inserted in the upper small bowel

Tubigrip – a type of tubular bandage

Tumble-form chair – a foam-moulded chair that helps children with special needs to develop postural control and encourage balanced weight-bearing

Valium – a brand of diazepam

Vallergan – an antihistamine

Webril – a brand of dressing/padding

acknowledgements

Stories are given life by the people who read them, so, to each of our readers, thank you for following our story. We hoped that, by giving you a seat on the roller coaster, you would obtain some appreciation of what a family goes through after a catastrophic event. For us, it's a roller coaster we can't get off. For you, whatever your situation, we hope you will be able to take from it one small thing that could change your life.

To Sally Collings, we say a big thank you for caring and piecing together sometimes fragmented words so they conveyed our true meaning. To Kevin O'Brien, Alison Urquhart and all at Random House, thanks for giving us a voice and the opportunity to preserve our diaries for posterity for Sophie, Mitchell, our extended family and all who read this book.

To our friends, both old and new, you played (and still do play) an integral part in our lives, which have been transformed forever. Thank you! Some friends have moved on and some are still there to lend a hand, both personally and for our charity, The Day of Difference Foundation. We are humbled by your support. To the wonderful people we have met along this journey, you have changed our thinking and given us a new understanding of the simple act of kindness.

To Mum, Dad, Ann-Louise and Gregory, thanks for being around when I needed you most. To my beautiful children, Mitchell and Sophie, I am so lucky to have your inspiration daily. Heartfelt thanks also to John and Catherine and the Delezio family.

To Ron, whose direct approach works well in a time of crisis, thanks for being such a great advocate. When it came to matters of life and death, everyone knew where you stood. I love you and thank you for your commitment to making changes for the better in so many areas.

To our medical teams, the hospital administration and volunteers, never underestimate the impact each of you have on a family. One act, one comment, can last a lifetime. Thank you for your dedication and commitment to our young.

Carolyn Martin

To my wonderful wife, Carolyn, thank God you are Sophie's mum, as Sophie needed a very special kind of care that only you could provide. There were times when your softness was exactly what Sophie needed, and other times when I saw the need of the protecting hand of her father.

I acknowledge all of the other parents that were and still are experiencing their own family trauma, especially the single parents, who do not have a partner to share the load.

I would also like to acknowledge the love and dedication of all of the medical staff in our children's hospitals and reflect on the fact that the so-called hardened professionals who work tirelessly saving our children are also mums and dads with sons and daughters, who get deeply affected by the job at hand. Seeing that Intensive Care doctor walking through the door crying before our meetings to discuss our daughter's future, the nurses who were not rostered on Sophie's operations due to the emotional strain, has shown us the human side that most people do not realise underlies their professionalism. It is also important to acknowledge the administration of the hospitals, especially the CEOs, who work tirelessly in organising a workforce of thousands, finding funding not only to open new facilities but also to raise the money necessary just to keep wards open.

Through our own experiences of operating our charity, The Day of Difference Foundation, we fully appreciate the commitment to the community demonstrated by the many thousands of charities that raise money so that our children can have the best possible chances in life. We would therefore like to express our gratitude to all of the children's charities in Australia, and those who volunteer for them and donate to them. Without you, many children would not survive their terrible traumas.

Let me also thank you, the reader, for caring enough about what happens to so many thousands of families around Australia every year, and for making your donation to the Day of Difference Foundation through your purchase of this book.

Ron Delezio